THE HOSPITALIZED CHILD AND HIS FAMILY

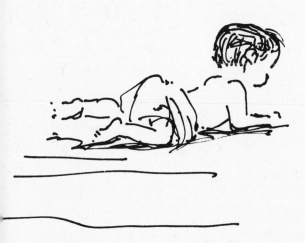

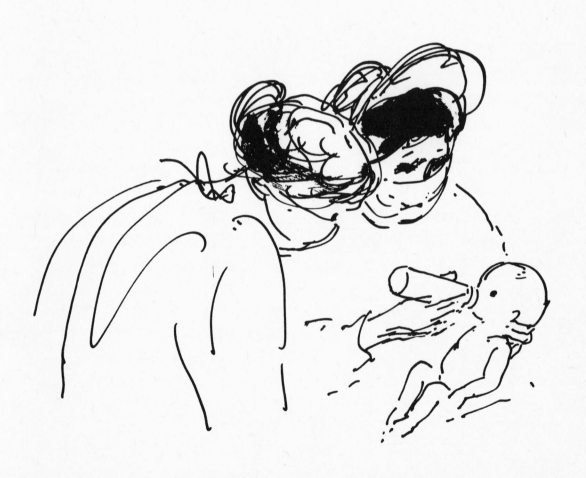

THE HOSPITALIZED CHILD AND HIS FAMILY

Editor: *J. Alex Haller, Jr., M.D.*
Associate Editors: *James L. Talbert, M.D.*
Robert H. Dombro, M.A.

Illustrated by Aaron Sopher

The Johns Hopkins Press: Baltimore

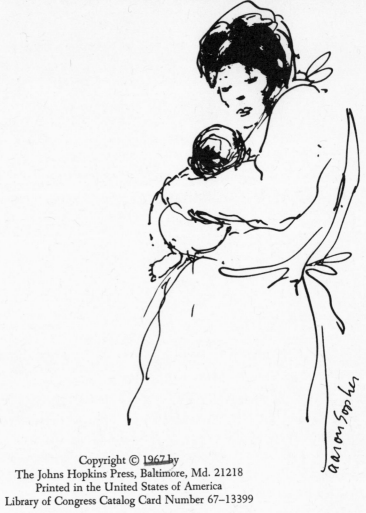

PREFACE

Physicians and nurses have always been intimately involved in the hospital care of sick children, but only rarely have they shown an active interest in anything beyond the child's physical and therapeutic needs. Usually the "other" aspects of hospitalization have been provided almost on an accessory basis by overburdened hospital personnel. It was from a common realization of this fact and from a growing concern with the total impact of hospitalization on a child that the idea arose for a multidirectional discussion of a child's relationship to and interreaction with his hospital environment.

As this idea developed within a small group of physicians, it became increasingly apparent that there were several of us in different specialty areas in the Children's Medical and Surgical Center of The Johns Hopkins Hospital who had been independently considering good and bad features of our common unplanned hospitalizations for children. Early in our discussions one physician stated his conviction that no adult remembered childhood hospitalization as a pleasant one! A wider sampling of physicians indicated an almost unanimous confirmation of this disturbing observation. In spite of the fact that there had been time for perspective and adult insight, there were only an isolated few who could honestly call their childhood hospital experiences either worth while or pleasant.

These hospitalizations had varied greatly in length of stay and severity of illness. In addition, the physicians' memory of the details had unquestionably been colored by their subsequent medical training and by their treatment of hospitalized children. Certainly hospital environments have changed greatly, both qualitatively and quantitatively, in the past three decades. Yet when the deficiencies in the childhood hospital experiences of these physicians were compared with the ones we considered significant, the remarkable feature was not the dissimilarities that might logically have been expected but rather the almost identical deficiencies and problems that have persisted. In many respects, therefore, many of us were able to discuss on a personal as well as a professional basis the complex features that constitute the total impact of hospitalization on a young child.

From the outset it has been our purpose to express these ideas in terms understandable to parents and yet technically accurate enough to stimulate nurses, paramedical personnel, and physicians in training. We gratefully acknowledge that many of the concepts are not original, but we believe that their correlation and personal interpretation by a group of concerned physicians are unique. If there is merit to this collection of thoughts, it is because they have come from the wide personal experience of physicians who have seen different aspects of hospitalization because of their divergent pediatric specialties.

The most helpful advice in the formulation of our final discussion topics and format came from Mr. Robert Dombro and his associates in the Child Life Program. As will be obvious from Mr. Dombro's description of the goals of the Child Life Program in Chapter VII, this exciting experiment is an attempt to provide an organizational structure for the co-ordination and implementation of many of the ideas discussed in the essays that follow. Theirs is one of a few full-time programs dedicated to making a child's hospital environment as much like a good home as possible. Out of the Child Life Program's evaluation of deficiencies in the child's hospital experiences and our own professional and personal observations, the original idea of a loose-knit series of discussions has come to fruition as a group of informal essays on the hospitalized child and his family.

These six essays do not constitute a closed circle of ideas; rather we hope they will serve as an interrelated series of discussions which will constitute a framework upon which to build correlated programs designed to improve a child's hospital experience.

J. Alex Haller, Jr., M.D.

CONTENTS

THE HOSPITALIZED CHILD AND HIS FAMILY

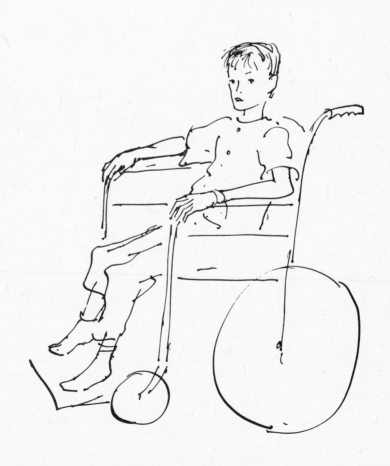

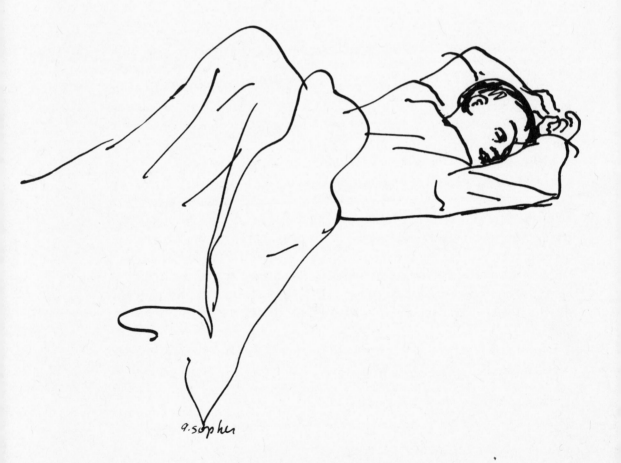

Chapter I

EFFECTS OF HOSPITALIZATION UPON THE CHILD

*Robert E. Cooke, M.D.**

I would like to attribute my interest in this problem to three people: Dr. Grover Powers, who was my professor at Yale and the reason why I am a pediatrician rather than a surgeon; Dr. Edith Jackson, a pioneer in the rooming-in movement and responsible for its popularity in hospitals throughout the country; and Dr. Milton Senn, who has maintained a strong interest in the problems of the hospitalized child.

Major interest in the effect of hospitalization on the child has come from psychiatrists as a result of clinical problems originating as residuals of hospitalization—namely, psychic trauma of the child. Prospective studies on the effects of hospitalization on children who have not yet developed difficulties have also revealed important results, which will be discussed subsequently. Even so, the question remains: Are the psychic injuries of hospitalization of sufficient importance to justify major efforts at prevention? The answer to this would have to be yes. The problem is a significant one with many facets that still require scientific investigation and, in addition, some direct application of knowledge we now have.

Interest in the effects of hospitalization are not new. One of the pioneers of pediatrics in Baltimore, Dr. Mason Knox, was interested in the problem of

* Given Foundation Professor of Pediatrics.

hospitalism in the institutions in Baltimore at the turn of the century.[1] These institutions, it is fair to say, were not modern hospitals by any means, but rather were foundling homes or chronic hospitals. His studies showed that an infant who remained in such a home or hospital for a period of a year had about nine chances in ten of dying during that year. That is, the mortality was about 90 per cent.

The causes for these deaths were many: respiratory infection, skin infection, diarrheal disease, and so forth. However, it was felt that there was much more to the problem than exposure to infectious agents. In addition, much was missing in the environment which was essential for the well-being of these babies. The 10 per cent in Dr. Knox's study who survived were those who were taken out of the institution for brief periods of time. He felt at that time that the change in environment, what we would now term the provision of attention and affection, made the difference.

Since those days of diarrhea and malnutrition and rickets there have been a number of studies that confirm the hazards of chronic hospitalization. In Teheran, for example, babies reared in orphanages have been compared with those cared for at home or in foster homes, and there were marked differences in rate of development—even in the quality of development (that is, the kinds of things which babies did)—in the two situations.[2] The study that is best known but, unfortunately, the least well controlled, was that of Spitz,[3] who demonstrated that babies in large orphanages, who were essentially without mothering, lacked attention, and were left to lie quietly in their cribs, had, in addition to poor physical growth and development, rather severe disturbances in affect which persisted for a long period of time. These problems were considered so serious that on some hospital services in this country and Europe personnel were assigned simply to hold the babies in order to give them the kind of attention they would receive at home. When a baby was not gaining weight, someone was assigned the job of restoring his emotional health. Reportedly the effect was often to produce a rapid improvement in weight gain and to cause associated minor illnesses to disappear.

[1] J. H. Mason Knox, Jr., "The care of institutional infants outside of institutions," *American Association for Study and Prevention of Infant Mortality. Transactions,* V (1914), 133.

[2] W. Dennis and P. Najarian, "Infant development under environmental handicap," *Psychological Monographs,* LXXI (1957), 60.

[3] R. A. Spitz, "Hospitalism: A follow-up report," *The Psychoanalytic Study of the Child,* ed. R. S. Eissler *et al.* (21 vols.; New York: International Universities Press, Inc., 1946), II, 113–17.

More recently there have been many studies concerning children who remain in the hospital not for periods of months but rather for days or even hours. These acute studies have tended to replace those made in the orphanages. I think they provide the answer to the question: Is psychic trauma of hospitalization a real problem?

In a prospective analysis of some 124 children who were being subjected to tonsillectomy, 25 of the group, or 20 per cent, had relatively severe residual emotional disturbances. Jessner *et al.*[4] also studied sixty tonsillectomy and adenoidectomy patients during the brief period of hospitalization and for several months thereafter. Initially twenty-eight appeared well adjusted to the hospital, but later this number decreased to only fifteen. Nineteen of the sixty displayed moderately poor adjustments in the hospital, with many residual fears and phobias, while thirteen were very poorly adjusted and developed major emotional difficulties. Prugh *et al.*[5] studied over 200 children divided into two groups and concluded that 60 in the control group had real problems of adaptation three months after hospitalization. A number of these reactions were severe.

There is good evidence in the literature, then, that we are dealing with an important problem. Indeed, the statement has been made that dangers of psychic trauma after minor surgery are considerably greater than the dangers of hemorrhage or infection. In most hospitals physicians have focused their attention on hemorrhage and infection and paid relatively little heed to the psychic disturbances of medical and surgical therapy.

One might legitimately ask why between 20 and 60 per cent of children have difficulties. I shall make an attempt somewhat artificially and pedantically to break the problem into separate elements with the hope that some facets may be correctable. It may be possible to minimize the difficulty if we can understand what these elements are.

Table I-1 is an attempt to explain the changes experienced during hospitalization. These are all changes in the environment and in the self to which adjustments must be made. I have broken them up into nonspecific changes that are not unique for the hospital and specific ones that are. I think all of us must realize that the major disturbance a child suffers is separation, which may be

[4] L. Jessner, G. E. Blom, and S. Waldfogel, "Emotional implications of tonsillectomy and adenoidectomy on children," *ibid.*, VIII, 126–29.
[5] D. G. Prugh *et al.*, "A study of the emotional reaction of children and families to hospitalization and illness," *American Journal of Orthopsychiatry*, XXIII (1953), 70.

divided into separation from things he is used to—home and furnishings, particularly his toys—and separation from people. Charlie Brown's friend Linus with his "sleepy" blanket is a splendid example of the former.

TABLE I-1

CHANGES REQUIRING ADJUSTMENT

I. Nonspecific (not unique for hospital)
   A. Separation from:
      1. Things—home and furnishings, toys
      2. Activities—school, play
      3. People—mother, father, siblings, friends
   B. Introduction to:
      1. New things
      2. New activities
      3. New people

II. Specific (unique for hospital)
   A. Separation complicated by:
      1. Illness
      2. Anxiety without outlet
      3. Suddenness
   B. Introduction to:
      1. Things—apparatus
      2. Activities—routines, procedures (painful or otherwise), meals, baths
      3. People—nurses, doctors, others (in large numbers)

The child who goes to summer camp also has a separation problem. Anyone who has worked as a counselor in a boys' camp observes the same problems as in hospitalization. When I was a first-year medical student, I was a counselor for a four-year-old and about eight five-year-olds. I encountered all types of regressive behavior—which is a nice way of saying that the boys were wetting their beds regularly. This can present quite a dilemma on a camping trip. Since sleeping bags are hard to ventilate, I spent most of the night watching those delightful separation problems.

The child over seven or eight loses contact, even during brief periods of hospitalization, with what seems to be the most important thing in his environment, namely school. He is separated from familiar people, above all from his mother. Although fathers often seem not to count a great deal, for certain age groups he is a very important person. Separation from him can be felt extremely, and I think that any program of care for children should provide opportunity for both father and mother to room in. The loss of siblings, the separation from friends—these are separations that occur if the child goes to camp or to visit his grandmother. In the hospital, however, we have also to consider the anxieties generated by exposure to new things—new activities and new people. All of you have entertained, and you remember that the first time is much more difficult than the second or third. You just do not know what to expect at first. The same is certainly true of any child who is hospitalized or goes to any other strange environment. The adjustment can at times be difficult.

What is the relationship of separation to hospitalization? How does it differ from going to camp or going to visit grandmother? The differences have to be considered in planning any program to minimize the effects of hospitalization.

First, separation is complicated by illness. Therefore the child is probably not as adaptable as he would be if he were feeling well. Unfortunately, we cannot obviate this factor except in elective admissions. Illness is a problem that we simply have to face up to as a severe complication of separation. It is interesting that since illness may render the experience an unpleasant one, it is one of the prohibitions against a child going to camp. Obviously, the way to prevent hospitalization problems is to do away with illness, but this is one solution that continues to escape us.

Another difficulty in the hospital is the anxiety generated by being in a new place and by the limitations on movement and illness by its very nature usually limits physical activity significantly. There is good evidence that physical activity is one of the ways of at least temporarily dissipating anxiety. Thus to restrict a child, admitted for an elective procedure, to bed is unsound not only from the physiologic standpoint but from the psychologic as well. Space for active physical exertion for elective admissions should be built into hospitals. The opportunity to roughhouse, to run around, to get rid of some steam, so to speak, is important and of great value.

The second element that renders hospitalization so different from visits to camp or to Grandma is the suddenness of the episode. This is as true for the child who is to be admitted for an elective hospitalization and ends up in the hospital, having been told he was being taken to the movies. The hospital is not exactly a movie house and such an introduction serves only to magnify the child's fears. The effect of such experiences is very different from that of the planned admission.

Finally, we must consider the absolute strangeness of the hospital environment. The child who may have a separation problem and who is somewhat limited because of his illness is exposed to situations that form the most frequent source of major problems in adjustment. Some of these situations can be terrifying to the child. Modern exposure to television medicine does little to impart a sense of security to the child when he learns that he must come to the hospital. In the horror movies I used to see—and I am told by the children of today that there are similar movies, only far better—the apparatus that created monsters looked just like the image intensifier in the X-ray Department. In fact, the producers might have saved money if they had done the filming in the X-ray Department. Efforts should be made to induce manufacturers to redesign their equipment —or some of it could be concealed or decorated—so that the hospital does not resemble a chamber of horrors.

Certainly hospitals and physicians should give the same thought to a problem dentists have solved so successfully. In the old days, when a patient walked into the dentist's office he was forced to look at all the things with which he would be attacked. The modern approach is to wait until his head is back and then to push a button that brings all the instruments into view. It is a much more civilized approach. It does not completely subdue the fear of having a tooth drilled, but it is psychologically sounder than having the patient collapse in the chair from fear after looking at all the instruments.

Unfortunately, hospitals are not always so enlightened. One of the real achievements in the Children's Medical and Surgical Center has been the elimination of all sorts of odd-looking apparatus from the corridors.

The introduction of the child to the unusual activities of the hospital comprises another important aspect of management. One should attempt to make the activities and routines as similar as possible to those the child has experienced at home. This is a big order with so many kinds of patients, yet there can be a certain reasonableness in the creation of routine. Sometimes it seems that great originality has been expended to make the hospital routine as unlike the home environment as possible. The nurse may still awaken you at five-thirty in the morning—when you had just fallen asleep—subject you to the thermometer and blood pressure routine, and then—when you are fully awake—arrive hours later with breakfast in an unattractive container. This situation has improved, but we still have a long way to go in planning routines. If routines cannot be changed, at least we should appreciate how different they are from home. For teenagers a day beginning at six-thirty in the morning is quite different from the schedule he maintains during weekends or vacation. In addition, all kinds of thoughtful ways are provided to awaken the patient. Breakfast may be withheld for certain blood drawing, so that as the patient awakens and reaches an elevated level of consciousness, someone enters to put a tourniquet around his arm, insert a needle, and draw out a "pint" of blood. Many of these activities may be necessary, but we must constantly ask how important they are for the individual patient.

How different is the routine of the Children's Medical and Surgical Center from what most children experience. The child awakes or is awakened between seven-thirty and eight and may be given medications and treatments such as compresses and vena puncture by the nurse or doctor. The food cart arrives shortly after eight; the trays are brought to the bedside. If the child needs help with his breakfast, nursing personnel (an aide, technician, student, or graduate) is assigned to see that aid is provided. The child is bathed after breakfast. This is certainly different from what he is accustomed to, because bathing for children is not a daily event in most households. It may be important that a child in the hospital be bathed every day, but I am not sure that it is really appreciated by all of them or is even necessary. Likewise, a bath in bed may seem particularly strange. If the mother is living in, she will be encouraged to help with his bath. This may be the first time for some older child that the mother has helped him with a bath in years.

The most reasonable part of the routine and one that is different from most hospital procedure is that the child is allowed to go to the playroom or play-school-dining area about ten in the morning if the doctor has indicated that he is able to do so. If it is felt that he may not go to the play area for any reason, such as isolation because of infection, then a member of the Child Life Program visits the patient in his room and brings interesting things to do. Television is available in every room for children over two years of age and is a great help. Lunch is served at noon, family-style, in the dining area. The patient is then encouraged to go to his room for a rest hour.

Visiting hours for parents or friends are between ten and nine-thirty. This contrasts strongly with the days when parents came twice a week for a brief period of a half-hour or an hour. Afternoon playroom activities begin at three. At five dinner is served at tables in the playroom. Since the playroom closes at six, the patient returns to his room after supper. This last contrasts with the normal home environment, where most activities are just beginning at six.

Patients receive medications and treatments throughout the day as scheduled. They go to various parts of the hospital for tests such as X ray, blood work, physical therapy. They are prepared for bedtime and allowed to watch television until a reasonable hour. Except for necessary medications or treatment, they sleep uninterrupted through the night.

Is this like home? There are certain strange elements. The bed and several other items are familiar, but the routine is unusual to the child, and we must expect that he will not feel at home for the first few days. The attempt to make the hospital like home is certainly a reasonable one. I have reviewed these obvious facts because it is very easy to forget that trivial items such as temperatures every four hours for the child who really does not need it is not only a nuisance to the nursing staff but can render the child's adjustment to the hospital even more difficult.

A typical day for an infant is quite similar, but the restrictions are more in items of dress—gowns to protect the child from infection—and regularity of feeding schedules. Although this routine is reasonable and may prove optimal, there is room for still further improvement. For example, one cannot help but feel that often the doctor is not as efficient or thoughtful as he might be. Why string out the procedure of obtaining blood and specimens over a period of many days when a little forethought might make it possible for one vena puncture to suffice for five? This simply requires planning and the realization that no one, particularly a sick child who is frightened by the "big syringe and needle coming after him," likes to be stuck with a needle.

The greatest problem in adjusting to new faces is that there are so many people in the hospital environment. Obviously the best way to care for a child in the hospital would be to have a single individual to act as doctor and nurse and dietician—and be his particular friend. This is the situation at home. His mother does all these things. Labor laws, house staff rules, nursing associations, and so forth, all make it impossible to provide this kind of treatment for an individual child. The more that the mother and father can do, the better it is. The child is comforted by his parents, but a crowd can be frightening. Different people—and there are so many different people who must care for a child—can produce real anxiety. Everyone is his friend, but he really knows no one. Continuity is difficult to obtain when personnel are constantly changing with each shift of nurses.

Some of these people may seem especially strange to the child. The doctor has vivid connotations for many children. Interestingly, some of the questions asked of children and their parents in the Head Start Program were: What sort of an individual is the doctor? Is he someone who helped you or someone who did not help you? Who essentially hurt you? At the beginning of Head Start about 50 per cent of the children felt that the doctor was not someone who was there to help them. This disturbing reply is a rather chastening lesson.

Many children come to the hospital with the idea that the doctor is bad. I think in general they are happier about nurses, but doctors have been used for a long time as threats—"If you don't drink your milk, you'll get sick and we'll have to take you to the doctor and he'll give you needles." These threats are still heard and, unfortunately, create the impression that doctors exist for the sake of punishment.

The factors that alter the adjustment of the child must be carefully considered. Some of these forces are outside the child and some are within him. These are listed in Table I-2. The attitude of the parents toward hospitalization is the single most important factor: it creates the internal environment for the child and thereby influences his responses.

I think effort can be made to alter the feelings of parents toward hospitalization. We can prepare them, if not for the immediate hospitalization, then for the next time and the next child. This is where the staff, informational material, and the approach of the physician can make an enormous difference in whether or not the parents consider hospitalization to be a threatening or a helpful experience. Thus one of the best ways to aid the child is to produce a healthy attitude within the parents towards hospitalization.

TABLE I-2
FACTORS AFFECTING ADJUSTMENT

I. Exogenous
    A. Attitudes of parents
    B. Duration of hospitalization (deprivation)
    C. Quantity of hospital experiences
    D. Quality of hospital experiences

II. Endogenous
    A. Physical and personality characteristics (feedback)
    B. Attitudes of child (preparation)
    C. Ability to cope
        1. Age
        2. Intelligence
        3. Nature of illness
        4. Resilience

I think all of us who are parents and who have had sick children must also realize that the emotional approach of the parent may be greatly influenced by the specifics of the illness. I do not think there is anything more traumatic for a parent, for example, than to find his child convulsing. This is a terrifying experience, which is life-threatening, and parents in general already think of hospitals as places where they bring people to die. One must realize, therefore, that even the parent whose child is mildly ill may believe him severely ill—because he must go to the hospital. We cannot always expect maximum co-operation and maximum understanding under these circumstances. However, I think that with proper consideration the attitude of parents can be modified to the extent that they can assume an important place in the team that is working with the child.

The duration of hospitalization also makes a significant difference. Studies have shown clearly that the longer the hospitalization the greater is the chance of residual effects. Ignoring the greatly prolonged periods of institutionalization which are encountered in orphanages, for example, relatively shorter hospitalizations, or periods of immobilization in a cast, may severely restrict the child's contacts and produce evidence not only of emotional but also of intellectual deprivation.

The quantity of hospital experiences—by this I refer to how much the child has actually undergone in his hospitalization—is another important determinant of emotional response. The child who has two cardiac catheterizations, experiences a cardiac arrest during one of them, and then undergoes surgery is exposed to tremendous and unusual stress. At the time of admission we must always consider just how much the child is going to be put through and perhaps organize our efforts to concentrate on those children who will be subjected to a very heavy load of difficult hospital experiences. There are a limited number of nurses, Child Life Program staff, and doctors, and I think it is not unrealistic to recognize that some children need more attention than others.

Another important aspect is the quality of the hospital experience. How does the hospital itself handle emotional problems? What is the attitude and procedure of the personnel? What attempts have been made to minimize some of the exogenous factors of hospitalization? A study was made as mentioned of the frequency of severe reactions in 200 children. These children were studied carefully, by intensive investigations before admission to the hospital, by observation during their hospitalization, and by repeated visits for posthospitalization. The control and the experimental groups were comparable in size and age composition. The number of severe reactions in the control group was much greater than in the experimental group. There was little difference in the incidence of moderate reactions. The frequency of minimal reactions was considerably greater in the experimental than in the control series. The control group was visited once a week for two hours by the parents. There were no Child Life Programs, and children received "good, routine pediatric care." There was no difference in medical personnel. In the experimental group, parents were allowed to visit every day and some of them lived in. There were attempts at school and recreational play programs. These efforts were reflected in a very definite reduction in severe reactions. There were also differences between the younger children and the older ones in this series. The big difference, of course, was the increased frequency of severe reactions in the younger child.

Endogenous factors are also important; yet they may frequently be ignored. The physical and personal characteristics of the infant or child greatly influence emotional "feedback." The attractive, outgoing, good-looking child will obviously have a very different hospital experience from the ugly, withdrawn child because of the feedback he receives on the basis of his engaging appearance. This is a factor we have all noticed but tend to forget in the day-to-day operation of a unit. In a premature nursery, for example, it is frequently true that there are infants whom everyone obviously likes. There are other prematures that nobody goes near except to feed. These last poor creatures, who do not have the personality to generate some interest and thus get very little feedback, can have a very different hospital experience—even in a center that is exerting every effort to improve the child's psychic well-being.

The critical determinant of the child's reaction is that of his own attitude, and, as I have said, this depends largely on the attitudes of the parents. This attitude can be modified, I think, by proper preparation. It is probably true that the older child will need a more detailed and lengthy preparation. The younger child, because of his shorter interest span, can be prepared much closer to the actual time of hospitalization. To tell a three-year-old all the details 'of a tonsillectomy he is going to have in six or eight months is a waste of time and may even be harmful. A few days' preparation for the younger child and several days to weeks for the older would seem reasonable.

As far as other factors are concerned, the ability to cope with one's situation is important. What are some of the elements of this ability? The child's age is extremely critical. Studies on tonsillectomy and adenoidectomy cases reveal that the psychic trauma of tonsillectomy is much greater in children under the age of three or four than in children between seven and ten. Possibly these findings represent the greater ease with which psychic disturbance can be detected in the younger child, but I do not think so. I think that the older child, through age and experience, has developed powers of adjustment. Therefore, age must be respected in determining the question of elective surgery. The longer such a procedure can be postponed the better it may be, at least from the psychic standpoint.

The intelligence of the child is another variable. I have had considerable experience with retarded children. I stress to the parents and staff that what is difficult for the normal child is usually far more so for the child with limited intelligence. In my own experience, the hospitalized mentally retarded child is much better cared for by his parents than by the staff. It is difficult for the staff to understand the idiosyncracies of each handicapped child. The mentally retarded child requires special attention and great effort to try to keep his environment as much like home as possible, and particularly to preserve contact with his mother and father. Many retarded children, when hospitalized, immediately stop eating, stop drinking, and become sicker than they were. We need the parents very much to help with these special children.

The nature of the illness may make a considerable difference. I remember one striking example, a child with measles encephalitis who was admitted to the hospital unconscious. She knew little of what was happening during a fairly long period of coma and awakened more confused than Rip Van Winkle. She had a poor remembrance of how she got to the hospital and of what had happened during her stay. I think that some of the personality disorders of measles may not be solely the sequelae of encephalitis but represent instead severe psychic trauma due to the child's confusion at waking up during some stage of treatment.

It is possible for a child who is quite ill on admission, who undergoes surgery and returns from anesthesia, to look very different from the way he did before going to the operating room. He has a bandage, a painful incision, and perhaps drains and tubes as well. These things can make quite a difference, and it is important that they be considered in the whole reaction pattern of the child.

Finally, there is the child who has so much resilience that he seems to adjust to any insult and comes through it, if anything, better for the experience. It reminds me of a story of the Frenchman and Englishman who were in a disabled plane that was forced to circle the field for hours before getting its wheels down and landing safely. During this long period of trauma the Frenchman wept and was in a state of constant agitation and excitement. John Bull sat quiet and composed, apparently without concern. When the plane finally landed, however, and the passengers went home, John Bull was a wreck for a week, while the Frenchman went off for a delightful weekend in the country. I think this story is representative of the differences we may see in children. Why these differences occur is not known.

The effect of acute hospitalization produces recognizable reaction patterns in the child. A clinging child who hangs onto everyone who comes by may be a child with a great deal of insecurity. Attempts to brush him off rather than permitting him to cling may compound the injury. At times, we see the opposite reactions: hostility and withdrawal. Regressive behavior, such as a return to bed-wetting and thumb-sucking, is fairly common and needs no special emphasis. Aggressiveness in school-age children who really are angry with their environment will cause them to strike out at their parents or others who are close to them. Late manifestations take the form of night terrors—particularly dreams about being left alone in the dark or fear of the dark. These are troublesome and common residuals, and we must recognize that they represent psychic scars. How important these problems may be is not always apparent. Negativism is a common reaction of children going home after hospitalization. They simply refuse to do what their parents wish. The parents do not understand this attitude and can perpetuate the problem by harsh punishment.

All of these reaction patterns represent some manifestation of the psychic trauma of hospitalization. However, the child does not have to be hospitalized to suffer this kind of trauma. At Hopkins we have been very anxious to develop a separate emergency room service for children. The child does not have to be an inpatient to be exposed to difficult, highly emotional circumstances in a hospital. Patients visiting the clinic may have many such experiences; those treated in the emergency room, for example, frequently see ghastly sights.

I know a little girl who since coming to the emergency room for relatively minor lacerations has developed a terrifying fear of ambulances. While she was waiting in the adult emergency room, an ambulance roared up and delivered a woman, who was carried through the door on a stretcher. She promptly staggered to her feet and gushed blood from a stab wound in the chest all over this little girl. Similar sights, including drunks who have fallen down and suffered jagged lacerations of the scalp, are all common in the usual large hospital emergency room. To inflict this environment on children seems to me a needless and terrible exposure and one which may induce severe psychic trauma in a rather short period of time. Separate emergency facilities should be available for children in every large general hospital.

I shall refer only briefly to some of the effects of chronic hospitalization—hospitalism, depression, withdrawal, repetitive activity, poor weight gain, listless behavior, and so on (see Table I-3). There have been excellent studies that have shown quite clearly that chronic patients may develop limited capacities to give and receive affection. They will have limited abilities in abstract thinking, and there is good evidence that their intelligence levels may be lowered significantly as a result of exposure to this type of deprived environment.

TABLE I-3
SIGNS INDICATING EFFECTS OF CHRONIC HOSPITALIZATON

I. Early
    A. Depression, withdrawal
    B. Repetitive activity (head banging, etc.)
    C. Poor weight gain, listlessness
II. Late
    A. Limited affection
    B. Limited abstract thinking(?)
    C. Lowered I.Q.(?)

What solutions are available to us? I shall point out only a few of the more obvious ones. It is apparent that, if medically feasible, operations should be postponed until the child has reached the age of five or six. Even then those procedures should be postponed if there have been recent disrupting emotional experiences. This is something few of us consider. Has something serious happened at home? Has there been a severe dislocation in the family? Has there been a death or have the father and mother recently separated? Has the child been severely hurt or a new baby been born in the family?

Second, the preparation of the child is extremely important. While the child may not understand everything he is told, his fantasies about the hospital may be healthier if he receives a little accurate information. I think it is important that the doctor who will be particularly involved in the care of the child have some contact with him beforehand. I also think that it is helpful to a child to bring along familiar objects to the hospital—the most familiar, of course, being the mother and, sometimes, the father.

16

The question of duration of hospitalization is also of great pertinence. There seems to be a feeling among some authorities that a period of adjustment in the hospital for a day or so before an operation is desirable. However, these same authorities feel that it is best for the younger child to have everything done in one day. Since the young child will have great difficulty understanding extensive preparation, it may be better simply to get the job done.

Finally, I should like to suggest that an effort be made to keep hospital routines as flexible as possible. Insofar as possible, a close resemblance to home life should be created. Objects and activities that are familiar to the child should be retained. This would mean bringing the patient's school, or a substitute, to him. Such a school is maintained in the Children's Medical and Surgical Center. Every effort should be exerted by equipment manufacturers and hospital administrators to try to abolish sights and sounds that may be terrifying and that in most instances could be corrected by relatively minor alterations. There is no way of knowing how much we can obviate the psychic scars of hospitalization if these changes are accomplished. All the studies that have been done so far indicate that one can expect a rather significant decrease—that is, one-third to one-half as many children with emotional problems.

In conclusion, I believe such an effort is worth while. If we but appreciate the great significance of adequate preparation of the institution, the staff, the family, and the child for the creation of a happy and emotionally healthy hospitalization, proper steps will be taken to reduce the frequency of residual psychic damage.

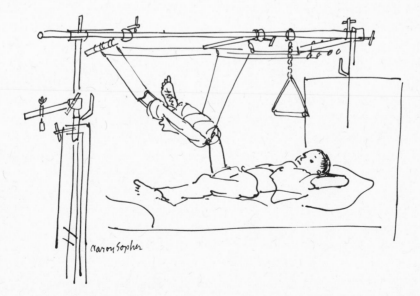

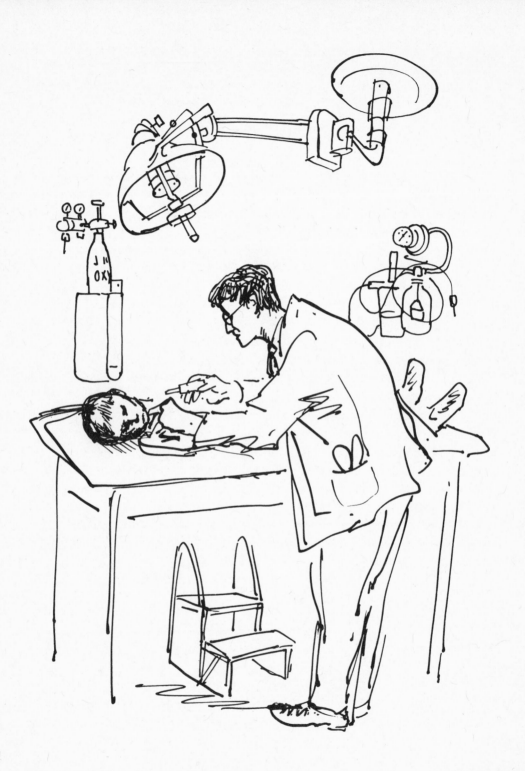

Chapter II

PREPARING A CHILD FOR HIS OPERATION

J. Alex Haller, Jr., M.D. *

What does an operation mean to a child? Without an answer we cannot intelligently prepare a child for this experience. Undergoing an operation or surgical experience presents a child with many threats and problems of emotional significance which are not usually present in a routine hospitalization. A careful, if not precise, description of this special hospital experience is necessary if we are to analyze its components.

An operation means an injury! Basically this constitutes both psychological and physiological trauma. Further, it is a controlled injury that occurs in an unfamiliar environment. All who have undergone trauma know that this is the poorest possible time to adjust to new emotional experiences. There is no worse time to relate to new people and new surroundings than immediately following an injury. Yet in the strange environment of a hospital, we are asking a child to undergo such trauma and at the same time to adjust to ancillary features.

Following an injury, the natural response of any animal is to escape from the immediate environment. A wounded creature will crawl to a secluded spot—his den or some hidden corner—and stay there until he has recovered. The opposite response is forced upon a child who undergoes an operation. He is exposed to a

* Associate Professor of Surgery, Children's Surgeon-In-Charge.

number of strange people and to a considerably different and unprotecting environment. In addition to these insults, white uniformed strangers visit him at irregular intervals. They poke at and examine him during this period of physical discomfort. These circumstances of course make natural animal behavior impossible.

Not many of us would hold a garden party or attempt a social gathering following an injury. Yet in many ways a hospital room duplicates these situations. Parents and friends descend upon the child following his operation. The patient has no alternative but to adjust to this emotional trauma that is unwittingly added to his physical discomfort!

Aside from the animal impulse to seek solitude and avoid exposure, there is another aspect of his trauma which may be of grave concern to the child. An operation is a *premeditated* injury. It may be obvious to the child that a period of prior thinking has taken place. Parenthetically, this element of premeditation carries with it the responsibility of using this period to prepare the child for his approaching operation. Of greater emotional consequence to the child is the fact that this premeditated injury is actually organized by his loved ones! The physicians and nurses are accomplices in this grand plot.

If the period prior to admission to the hospital is not used to prepare the child, his planned operation becomes in addition a *surprise* injury in the child's mind— a surprise into which he is led by his parents. There is perhaps no more trying emotional experience than sudden, unexpected trauma. If the child suspects any connection between his parents and the injury, this suspicion may create a far-reaching emotional impact on the relationship of the child with his parents. Stripped of adjectives and modifiers, these are stark statements. Yet they are essentially factual. An operation *is* an injury. Although none of us, regardless of his relationship to the patient, is going to allow this experience to be stripped of all adjectives and modifiers, such can be the impact upon the child unless there is careful prior explanation and emotional preparation.

Let us consider some of the ways in which hospitalization can become a wholesome experience. Many of these thoughts are themselves in a process of growth and development. Many of the published studies on the child's response to hospitalization concern children with relatively chronic admissions. The major problem in these instances has been deprivation of affection and love during the child's long separation from his home environment. We are discussing an entirely different type of hospitalization, one which is short-term and includes an operation.

20

The short-term hospital stay coupled with an operation has features significantly different from the long-term stay. The chronic hospitalization has its own problems and its own adjustments, but these result primarily from *omission*. Omissions of attention and affection can be corrected by bringing various specialized personnel, family members, and friends into the child's new environment.

The child who is admitted for a short-term hospitalization for an operative procedure, on the other hand, also has problems that result from *commission*. These must be recognized and their emotional consequences considered in some detail. The child is almost simultaneously committed to a strange environment, forced to undergo an uncomfortable operation, and required to relate to many strange people.

Thus the relationship of a child to the hospital will depend upon the length of time he stays in the hospital and the type of experience he has there. There are quantitative aspects of a hospital experience just as there are qualitative ones.

It must be remembered that a truly successful surgical procedure embodies far more than simply the correction of an abnormality or the relief of a diseased state. We have come to expect these results. To be truly successful, it must send home a child who is emotionally undamaged by his hospital stay. The surgeon is primarily concerned with removing the tonsils if they are diseased or the appendix if it is infected, but an operation is completely successful when a well child returns to his home environment and is the better for his hospital stay. His hospitalization should be a strengthening emotional experience. No event in the child's life is without effect on the course of his normal growth and development. No experience leaves us on the same plateau at which we found ourselves prior to it. A child will be changed in one way or the other from his trip to the hospital. An operation carries with it, therefore, the additional heavy responsibility of making it a worth-while experience.

An operative procedure during the child's hospitalization may be looked upon as an adventure. An adventure has considerable meaning to children, for they are very familiar with them from television and radio. They know that there are several classic ingredients to an adventure, and not all are pleasant. An adventurous life includes hardships and suffering, even for the hero. But basically the good guy always triumphs, and the Lone Ranger rides off with Tonto!

A child's experience in the hospital has exactly the same potential. There will be hardships and suffering, but as the hero of this adventure the child will go riding safely home, ready to face another exciting episode.

PREPARING THE CHILD AT HOME

In attempting to focus more precisely upon some aspects of a child's hospitalization, it might be useful to list some of the important influences that mold his experience before he arrives at the hospital. The key individuals in this experience are listed in Table II-1. Certainly the earliest and most important influence comes from his parents. To be a directing and thus helpful influence, the parents must first be made aware of the facts that relate to a child's hospitalization. This information must be precise and accurate in detail. Often parents attempt to prepare their child for a hospitalization and an operative procedure when they have faulty information and unfounded anxieties of their own. This background creates problems in terms of the parents' own concern and may make it extremely difficult for them to communicate to their child an accurate description of the experience he is about to undergo.

TABLE II-1
KEY INDIVIDUALS IN PREPARING CHILD FOR AN OPERATION

I. Parents

II. Pediatric nursing staff

III. Anesthesiologist

IV. Surgeon

An important by-product of acquiring accurate information about hospitalization is that the parents' own fears are allayed as they become aware of the events that lie ahead. Anyone who has experience in teaching realizes that no teacher is effective unless he knows his subject well. In the same way only informed parents can orient a child to a new experience or a new adventure.

In transmitting this information, parents must be able to present the facts in terms that will be not only understandable to the child but will also fulfill the emotional requirements and needs of their particular child. There are certain children to whom it is fairly easy to transmit information that will be helpful in their coming experience. There are other children to whom it is very difficult to get across even simple, factual information. Who should know better how to do this than the child's own parents? But they must be comfortable with the facts themselves before attempting to adapt them to the child's requirements.

Healthy anticipation is always an important part of any coming adventure or experience. The timing of the preparation for hospitalization is therefore of consequence to the child. No one knows exactly how long before the experience a given child should be told of it, but certain guidelines are helpful. It makes very little sense to give a detailed preparatory speech to a young child several weeks or months before it is to occur. The attention span of a child in the younger age group is quite short. He is not able to retain this type of information for more than a few days. A six-year-old boy will be excited all week about a football game with Dad, but several week's anticipation would be a useless eternity to him. Equally thoughtless is the parent who tells his child as he gets out of the automobile in front of the hospital that he is going to have an operation the next day. Neither approach is a proper preparation, but in general, the younger the child, the shorter the preparation period should be.

The adventure in the hospital should be presented to the child as a sequential one. This concept bears re-emphasis, because the important sequence of events is that the child is *at home,* he *goes to the hospital,* and then he *comes home again.* Many children know that other members of the family or neighbors have been admitted to the hospital. They are also aware of the fact that some people come to the hospital and die. They may have had personal experiences with a grandmother or with great-aunts who went to the hospital and did not come home. We must be certain in our discussion of the child's hospital adventure that we include this circular aspect of his experience.

Orientation of children may be achieved in a number of different ways. It is often helpful to read about another child whose hospitalization involves an operative procedure. Children like to hear stories, and they also find it very easy to put themselves into a story. Any anxiety the child may have can often be allayed in an impersonal way through the medium of a story about hospitalization. This technique is particularly suited to families where reading is a natural part of the day's activities.

One mild word of caution is in order in relation to story reading. Many children are inclined to consider all stories to be fantasies. Stories are not true events to them; they are all fairy tales. But within reason, a spritely story about hospitalization is often quite helpful.

Play-acting is another of the delights of childhood. It offers a real opportunity for becoming involved in an experience before it really occurs. This is true whether the child is playing Mother and Daddy or whether she is playing wedding or housekeeping. The important principle is that through play-acting children are able to pretest some of their emotional experiences before the actual event.

In this period of preparation, family participation is extremely important. A child depends upon other members of his family for all his experiences. Various types of minor injuries have occurred in the past, and the family was always there to provide emotional support and care. In discussing his operation, the fact that his whole family will be participating must be clearly communicated to him. It may be a vicarious participation in the sense that "Daddy will be outside the hospital most of the time, but he will be thinking about you," or, "Sister will have to stay home, but when you come back, you can tell her all about your hospital!" It is in this context of active participation by the family that rooming-in may play a vital bridging role between home and hospital and between hospital and home.

THE ROOMING-IN MOTHER AS A BRIDGE BETWEEN HOSPITAL AND HOME

Of all the hospital experiences that children must undergo, the short-term hospitalization that includes an operation is one in which the mother's rooming-in can play a most important role. It is unreasonable to expect a young child to relate to hospital personnel and to a new environment during a very short admission in which he is also undergoing an operation. If a child is hospitalized for two or three weeks for observation and treatment, he has time to establish some relationship with his doctors and nurses. In such an admission it is not nearly so important to have the emotional support of his mother. For example, a child who is admitted for a tonsillectomy or a hernia repair may be in the hospital for no longer than forty-eight hours. A living-in mother can be extremely helpful not only as an emotional support but also for the other important functions that she performs in his day-to-day care (see Chapter III). The various aspects of the parents' role in their child's operation are summarized in Table II-2.

PREPARING THE CHILD IN THE HOSPITAL

If the mother rooms in with her child or is able to visit frequently, she may play a significant part in the continuing preparation of the child in the hospital.

TABLE II-2

PREPARING THE CHILD FOR AN OPERATION
THE PARENTS' ROLE

I. Obtain precise, accurate information

    A. To allay own fears
    B. To adapt facts to individual needs of child

II. Transmit information with healthy anticipation

III. Plan sequential adventure (home—hospital—home)

    A. Reading
    B. Play-acting
    C. Family participation

IV. Rooming-in mothers

In most hospitals this is largely a nurse's role. It is a uniquely important one. There are a few guidelines that may make the nurses' task easier and more effective. The nurse must be a truthful guardian. Most children will relate warmly and spontaneously to a nurse who gives accurate and truthful information, but she must also show active concern for the child. When the admission blood tests are taken, the nurse should tell the child that he will have a needle prick that will hurt for just a moment and that she will be there with him. The child beyond infancy will accept brief uncomfortable treatment if it is presented as both a routine and an inevitable test and if he has the support of his friend. For the infant, speed and gentleness replace any explanation. A nurse must personify dependable security. Security is not a need that ceases after the trials of admission: it must be there the next day and the day following the operation. In an environment entirely strange to the child, it should be, in addition, a predictable security. This security is probably best engendered by attending to the child's routine needs, such as helping him unpack his hospital clothes and going with him to the playrooms and to the dining area. A student nurse or senior nurse's aide can ideally fulfill this role, and, if at all possible, a child should have one person assigned to him throughout the shift. This relationship should be maintained during his hospitalization even though several children will be assigned to one nurse or nurse substitute.

An effective nurse will also be a gentle guide during the orientation and preparation. Sometimes gentle guidance may seem practically impossible with a

25

distraught child, but a sincere attempt to win the child's confidence and to guide him through the routines of admission will pay rich dividends.

Finally, a nurse must be a consistent friend. One of the disturbing features of the usual relationship between nurse and patient is that the nurse brings the needles. This is an area in which paramedical personnel can be of great help. The consistent friend does not have to be a nurse. She may very well be a member of a Child Life Program or some similar group. There must be someone in this role to whom the child can relate. Preferably this relationship should not be destroyed from time to time by painful medication or uncomfortable therapy.

Hospital orientation and admission bring the child in direct contact with hospital routines that may vary widely. We still have a strong tendency to use adult forms of hospital routine and to try to adapt the child to them rather than vice versa. It makes no sense at all, for example, to wake a healthy child at midnight and at four in the morning to record his normal temperature. This is especially true for the well child who is scheduled for an early morning operative procedure. The nurse's rapport with the child during admission and hospital orientation will determine the success or failure of her preparation of the child for his operation.

The preoperative orientation of the child is one of the nurse's most important functions. The dress and appearance of the surgical personnel are different from other hospital personnel. Masks and gowns may carry certain mysterious connotations to the child. He is not accustomed to seeing a masked individual except one who is about to rob a bank or to harm someone. He is concerned about the masked people and those who wear special clothing around him. It is often easy to make a child feel at ease with these uniforms by having small gowns and masks that he can try on and parade before his fellow patients. Sometimes a mask or scrub cap on a favorite doll or animal will be a more acceptable way of making contact with these items. If he can be brought into contact with these components of a surgical environment *before* undergoing his operative procedure, he will be much better able to accept them. He will not look upon them as manufactured or instigated especially for or against him.

The same holds true for oxygen tents and a number of other machines that look threatening to a child. It is important that he be able to recognize them as a normal, standard part of the hospital environment. This relaxed familiarity can be achieved by allowing a child to come into contact with these objects during a period of relative security and in the absence of duress—in other words, before his operative procedure.

Figure 1 is a view of the Intensive Care Unit of the Children's Medical and Surgical Center. Any child or adult would be justifiably concerned if he suddenly opened his eyes and for the first time saw these machines looking down upon him. Not only do there appear to be eyes at the top of the blood pressure recorders, but below them there are a number of other threatening devices. When lights start blinking and noises erupt from this machine, it resembles closely a robot monster. Children are familiar with many weird types of mechanized toys, which are acceptable as part of their normal home environment because *they were introduced in this way*. But this will not be true of the hospital monsters if a machine that has no familiar reference to the care of the sick child suddenly appears.

The oxygen tent is a similar source of fear. To encase a child in any tent other than one associated with sleeping bags and camping out presents a clear threat to him. In the first place children do not like to be separated from their friends. But to be separated inside a closed sack that has something pumped into it immediately signifies that its occupant is being gassed. This is exactly the way a butterfly is put to sleep before it becomes a part of the child's insect collection. To prevent this interpretation every child who may possibly require increased humidity after anesthesia must be put into a tent before his operation. Older children can tuck down the tent flaps and younger ones may close the zippers as they play in and out of the practice tent. It is often more of a game if several children can learn about the oxygen tent together. If a child's mother is living in she must put her head inside, too. Familiarity may breed healthy contempt.

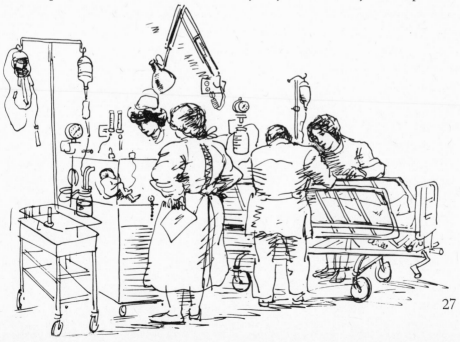

Only by allowing the child to come in contact with the recovery room environment before his operation can he be made to feel secure afterward. He must enter the oxygen tent accompanied by a friend, whoever she may be. Only in this way will he be able to accept this experience in the postoperative period without being terrified. These complex and vital aspects of the nurse's role in the child's hospitalization are summarized in Table II-3.

TABLE II-3

THE NURSE'S ROLE

I. As a truthful guardian

II. As a dependable security

III. As a gentle guide
    A. Admission routine
    B. Orientation
        1. Masks, gown
        2. Oxygen tents
        3. Machines

IV. As a consistent friend

It is important to mention the anesthesiologist's role in the child's operation, because it is one part of the child's operative experience which is least understood by many parents and certainly by most children. Being put to sleep in a hospital may carry fearful connotations to a child. Children know that many old people "just go to sleep and don't wake up." This is what the child is often told when his aunt dies. "Old Aunt Jane was very sick, she was taken to the hospital, and she just went to sleep and ended up in heaven." The child is not anxious to undergo a related experience. It is important to recognize this similarity and to emphasize to the child that sleep for an operation has a waking up, just the same as going to sleep at home is followed by waking up in the morning. For the school-age child it is often helpful to explain that he must be asleep so that he will feel no discomfort during his operation and will not be worried about what the doctors are doing and saying.

The anesthesiologist's role is at least twofold. In the first place he is responsible for a professional evaluation of the child's medical condition. This will naturally include in it any effects of prior hospital experiences upon the child. If he has had a fearful or unhappy experience with any kind of anesthesia, local or general, his impending trip to the operating room is a much greater threat to him.

The anesthesiologist's second task is to give a satisfactory anesthesia and yet avoid frightening the child. To accomplish this the anesthesiologist must know the child personally prior to putting him to sleep. Such a relationship can only be accomplished by a visit with the child in his own bedroom. It need not take much time, but it is important that the child be able to recognize the individual in the operating room who will accompany him through the anesthesia. This experience, too, may be looked upon as an adventure.

A tiny infant or very young child is not able to participate in an adventure story, but it is quite easy to involve an older child in a real adventure while he is undergoing anesthesia. Very young preschoolers are familiar with space travel and can usually be enthralled into helping to hold the anesthesia mask near their faces like a space pilot. The newer anesthesia gases are odorless, so the ether fear is no longer a problem. The blood pressure cuff is also standard equipment for an astronaut, so the first-grader may like to pump up his own cuff. The anesthesiologist must be ready for many questions from the older children if he makes the anesthesia a real adventure. Recently a nine-year-old was being prepared for orbit, but when the mask was lifted to his face he twisted his head, looked directly into the anesthesiologist's eyes, and said, "Wait a minute—what are the plans for re-entry?"

Premedication is a very significant part of the anesthesia. Ideally premedication in older children should permit co-operation and should completely alleviate apprehension. This goal is difficult to achieve, but it is a worthy one. The infant or the very young child need not co-operate when he arrives in the operating room. As a matter of fact, many anesthesiologists feel that it is best to give an infant under two heavy sedation so that he is practically asleep before the anesthesia is induced.

These are significant details, since the anesthesia may have more serious emotional aftereffects than the actual operation. If asked what part of a coming operative experience he dreads most, almost everyone will volunteer that it is *not* the postoperative pain but rather the anesthesia, the experience of being totally in the hands of another individual. This feeling is reflected also in the young child and should not be overlooked. The important contributions of the anesthesiologist are summarized in Table II-4.

The surgeon's preoperative role, in addition to his operative participation, is also an important one. He should have an opportunity for prehospitalization and preoperation discussions with the child and his parents. This implies that the

TABLE II-4

THE ANESTHESIOLOGIST'S ROLE

I. Professional evaluation

II. Personal acquaintance

III. An anesthesia adventure

surgeon has seen the child before he comes to the hospital. It also implies that the surgeon has met one or both parents before the child is admitted to the hospital and that he has discussed with them the facts of the operative procedure.

We have discussed the child's preoperative contact with the nurse in the area that will become his postoperative environment. The surgeon's participation is also important because he will be at the child's bedside in the postoperative period. Unless the surgeon is identified by the child with this environment *before* his operative procedure, he may be looked upon as a threatening stranger whose function is unclear.

A simple description of the aftereffects of the operation is of great value in cementing the child-surgeon relationship. It is not important to tell the child about the operation itself in great detail, but it is of greatest consequence to explain to the child how he is going to feel *afterward*. This may represent the most important aspect of the surgeon's relationship to the child. It is one thing to tell a child that he will have his tonsils removed, but to omit telling him that his throat will be very sore for several days leads the child to question the surgeon's honesty, if not his intentions. To describe the small incision that will repair his hernia is all very well, but to omit saying that his groin will hurt when he tries to walk is to leave the child with an incomplete description of the operative experience and to risk hearing him say to his mother, "That man hurt my stomach!"

A rapid return toward normal habits for a child should be a major goal of the surgeon. The sooner the child can recognize that he is no longer ill or incapacitated, the quicker he will recover from his operative experience. Prolonged use of intravenous fluids—even continuing to serve food to a child in bed—may convince the child that he is still quite sick. If a child is allowed to hop out of bed as soon as it is professionally indicated and allowed to visit, to be visited, to go to the playroom, and to eat normally in the playroom, he realizes that his illness is over.

The opportunity of mobilizing children rapidly and helping them return to normal habits is one of the significant ideas that are being incorporated in new hospital architecture. Multipurpose playrooms are used for a dining area, as well as for school and play. This is one of the most attractive features of the new Children's Medical and Surgical Center in The Johns Hopkins Hospital. If food is available and a picnic is going on in an attractive playroom, a child who has had a hernia operation in the morning is anxious to be up that afternoon to join his friends for supper. He does not want to be excluded from this event because it was a normal part of his preoperative experience. He became used to it in the short but important period of hospitalization prior to his operation. The sooner it can be recognized that the child is not seriously ill (the surgeon's recognition of this is best communicated to the child by allowing him a normal routine), the better and more quickly he will be able to carry out his usual activities.

The surgeon's role thus begins in the home and continues until the child is returned to his home. The facets of his contribution are outlined in Table II-5.

TABLE II-5
THE SURGEON'S ROLE

I. Prehospitalization discussion (child and parents)

II. Preoperative contact in the hospital

III. Simple description of aftereffects of operation

IV. Rapid return toward normal routine (visiting, eating, playing)

In preparing a child for his operation, then, we must first attempt to understand its full significance for him. From this sound basis we can lead the child into his new adventure. The surgeon's initial role is to present realistically to the parents the facts of hospitalization. They in turn can orient their child, for each child is a unique individual. His experience can be planned most logically by informed parents who know their child and are able to predict and evaluate his responses. The hospital personnel supplement this home preparation by showing a child the hospital environment that is their professional home.

We can rest assured that a child will trust those who are patient and truthful with him. He can be told with honesty that an operative experience is an adventure. He can be lead excitingly into this experience, for adventure is a basic ingredient of childhood. To the properly prepared child, it can be truly high adventure—if we help to make it so.

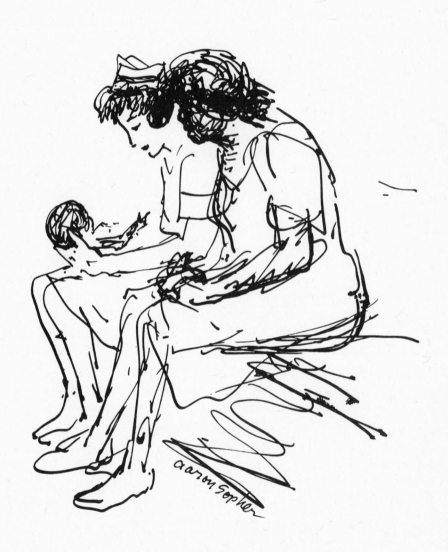

Chapter III

ADVANTAGES OF MOTHER LIVING IN WITH HER HOSPITALIZED CHILD

*Alexander J. Schaffer, M.D.**

A recent personal experience reminded me, once again, of the necessity for continued emphasis on this subject. I was responsible for leading a round table on the management of patients in hospital. One of the topics I presented for consideration was "What Is the Parent's Role in the Hospital?"

During the course of the discussion I asked for a show of hands to indicate the number of physicians present whose own pediatric departments permitted mothers to live in with their children. There were about sixty pediatricians in the room, and I was amazed to find that only five or six hands, perhaps seven, were raised. Why do we have so much difficulty getting this concept across to the pediatricians of this country and, through them, to their paramedical and lay associates?

I think the problem stems first from a lack of knowledge of the facts, and second from a lack of empathy—that is, from an inability to project oneself into the skin of another person. This is especially difficult if that person is totally different from you, if, for example, he or she is much smaller and much younger. Our first task is to ascertain the facts insofar as we possibly can for all ages and for all conditions of children being hospitalized, and our second is to establish a course of action based on those facts. Once we have laid out this course of action we must not let considerations of minor importance stand in the way of

* Associate Professor of Pediatrics.

carrying out what we consider to be ideal methods of handling children in the hospital.

What are the facts? Can we speak with any certainty concerning the effect on children of sojourns in hospitals?

Separation of children from their mothers is a relatively recent phenomenon. No primitive people permit it. I had some experience with this twenty years ago when I was stationed in Fiji during World War II. In Suva, the capital, there is a big, well-equipped hospital. In those days the children's ward did not present a row of beds, each containing a child. One saw instead groups of families around children. The mother was there always, often a couple of aunts, a grandmother or two, and much of the time the father. Each family had its own cooking utensils, and in the middle of the stone-floored ward they cooked the foods to which their children were accustomed. This is particularly important in Fiji, since in this group of islands Fijians comprise about half the population; the other half are East Indians who were brought over as indentured servants and stayed on. Fijian mothers cooked fish and breadfruit and taro root for their children, and Indian mothers made rice dishes for their children. The children's families were there, their accustomed food was there, and there was always someone nearby to do things for the child as he had had them done for him at home. In the jungles of Africa, in Lambaréné, Albert Schweitzer found it necessary to permit families to be present in the same way.

Folklore can be very deceptive, but one must not forget that it gave medicine foxglove, quinine, and ephedrine, among other invaluable drugs. There may indeed be some validity to folklore. Until the late modern era it was considered unthinkable to place a young child in hospital without his mother. Robertson[1] tells us that in the 1700s an act was proposed to Parliament recommending that a children's hospital be constructed. A report of a committee to Commons contained this statement: "A very little reflection will clearly convince any thinking person that such a scheme can never be executed. If you take away a sick child from its parents or its nurse, you break its heart immediately." This statement is not necessarily invalid because it is stated in nonscientific terms.

When we entered the twentieth century, pediatrics began to be a science, and the growth of scientific knowledge was soon phenomenal. We became more and more deeply interested in organic disease, in the structural defects of organs, and in metabolic disorders, and we equated illness with these concrete things. Illness equals cirrhosis of the liver, or rheumatic disease of the heart, or rickets,

---

[1] J. Robertson, *Young Children in Hospitals* (New York: 1958).

and so on. We thought of illness in terms of external assaults on the child by viruses, bacteria, fungi, poisons, or in terms of nutritional deficiencies. We focused so sharply on the sick organ and the disease process that we fragmented the child into a group of organs and systems and forgot entirely to keep looking at the whole child. It was in this period when we were so interested in what was happening physically and chemically to our little patients that we decided that mother was dispensable. The upshot was that when I became an intern in the early twenties, mothers were allowed to visit their children once a week, no matter how short or how long their hospital stay. Parents could remain for all of two hours! We were taught mothers were dangerous as carriers of infection and that frequent visits delayed "settling down" in the hospital.

Soon thereafter—and this brings us into the 1930s—we began to reap some of the seeds we had sown. It became widely recognized all over the country that some children did not do well when they were confined to the hospital for short periods, and they did even worse when they were confined for long periods. We began to recognize a syndrome that we called "hospitalism." "Hospitalism" was a disorder in which the child, although he may have eaten well, failed to gain weight and often failed to grow in height. His intellectual development was retarded and his personality changed for the worse in various ways. We saw the same syndrome develop in orphan asylums and in bad foster homes, and more recently we have even seen it evolve within the home. For this reason we now call it "maternal deprivation" or "parental deprivation" rather than "hospitalism." The disease was described and pediatricians read about it in various journals, but in the main it was ignored. A few warm-hearted men blessed with empathy paid attention to it, like Grover Powers in New Haven. These men initiated trials of methods whereby hospitalism might be prevented or reduced in intensity. It was at this time that a program of TLC (Tender Loving Care) was first tried as a prophylactic measure. This was unquestionably a great help. But was it enough?

With increased awareness of the problem and with the birth of a new specialty, child psychiatry, there began an era of scientific study of the problem. In spite of the deficiencies of some of these early studies, they were useful to us. Perhaps one of the most important was the one by Dane Prugh[2] at the Childrens Medical Center in Boston. Prugh and his associates studied 100 children who had been admitted to the hospital under their old plan, which was exactly like the plan in the Harriet Lane Home when I was a house officer. Mothers were

[2] D. G. Prugh *et al.*, "A study of the emotional reactions of children and families to hospitalization and illness," *American Journal of Orthopsychiatry,* XXIII (1953), 70–106.

allowed to visit once a week for two hours, and there were no provisions for play, study, or any kind of extra attention for the child. Prugh then admitted 100 children and treated them in a way which in that era seemed enlightened and compassionate. He had them prepared before they came into the hospital by talks from their own physicians and from members of his department. He allowed the mothers to visit once a day. He had a good play program set up for them, and a child psychiatrist supported each child by talking to him every other day during his stay in the hospital.

How much did Dr. Prugh accomplish by his enlightened handling of hospitalized children? He found that under the old impersonal system 92 out of 100 children showed some kind of emotional disturbance when examined one or two weeks after discharge. In the enlightened treatment group this figure dropped to sixty-eight. Three months later 60 per cent of the control group still showed some emotional disturbance, versus 44 per cent of the experimental group. Overall, something had been accomplished by instituting measures to make the child's stay more pleasant and more comprehensible to him.

In the experimental group 14 per cent exhibited severe reactions, and adverse behavior persisted in about half of these for three months or more. When the total group was split into various age groups, it became clear that for children three years old or less, enlightened care had not done much good at all. There were severe reactions in 50 per cent of the control group and in 44 per cent of the experimental group of this age. By severe reactions I mean overt and serious upsets in personality and behavior. These included night terrors, and increased dependence manifested by constant clinging to the mother and by refusal to let mother leave the house. Manifestations of regression were not infrequent. Children who had long before learned to control their bladder and bowel functions regressed to the point where they wet or soiled the bed or began to suck their thumbs or to masturbate. Some of them responded by fits of anger, combativeness, and destructiveness. A 14 per cent over-all severe reaction rate, even under good care, and a 44 per cent severe reaction rate in children three years and younger is hardly an ideal outcome.

There were other good studies. David Levy's,[3] one of the earliest ones, illustrates the influence of age. His was a retrospective study and was not controlled, but the results fit well with those of many others. He concluded that about half of the children in the zero to one-year-old group had severe reactions (there were not enough cases to hazard an estimate of percentage); of the one-to-two-year-

[3] D. M. Levy, "Psychic Trauma of Operations in Children," *American Journal of Diseases of Children*, LXIX (1965), 7–25.

olds, 58 per cent had severe reactions; of the two-to-three-year-olds, 33 percent; of the three-to-four-year-olds, 16 per cent; and of the four-to-twelve-year-olds, 9 per cent. We commonly say now that this is not a disorder that affects older children, but if one out of ten or eleven older children are disturbed by hospitalization, we surely ought not to think of it as being confined to the younger age group.

Someone was bound sooner or later to come up with the ultimate in controlled experiments. Sipowicz and Vernon,[4] at the Children's Memorial Hospital of Chicago, studied twenty-four pairs of twins, one of whom had been hospitalized, the other not. They found that sixteen of the twenty-four hospitalized twins developed emotional disturbances. This finding was most marked in the six-month-to-four-year-old age group.

I shall not discuss those studies that focused on the effects of long-term hospital stay. Many of these children fare as poorly as those who are confined to orphan asylums or raised in unhappy foster homes.[5] Some of them are harmed for life, left in a state that closely resembles that of a brain-damaged child. They are hyperactive, have personality disorders, can no longer make close attachments with any one individual, and demonstrate inability to concentrate or to learn. Many of them develop into psychopathic personalities who cannot tell the difference between right and wrong.

So much for these negative studies. There have been a few positive all-out trials made by pediatricians or child psychiatrists who were thoroughly dissatisfied with the results of conventional hospital care. The first of these with which I am familiar was made by Sir James Spence in England. Sir James had observed the reactions of children to hospitalization in England for a number of years; when he came to the United States to work with the great Dr. Howland, he saw the same results. Shortly after he returned to England he became a professor with a hospital of his own in Newcastle-upon-Tyne, and there he almost immediately set into operation a living-in program. A few years later he was asked to deliver the Sir Charles West Lecture,[6] an annual event of great pediatric importance. He used as the subject for his address his experiment of mothers' living in. The lecture was an all-out endorsement of the virtues of living in and a plea that it be used more widely.

[4] R. R. Sipowicz and D. T. A. Vernon, "Psychological Responses of Children to Hospitalization," *ibid.,* CIX (1965), 228–31.
[5] W. Goldfarb, "Psychological privation in infancy and subsequent adjustment," *American Journal of Orthopsychiatry,* XV (1945), 247–55.
[6] J. C. Spence, "The Care of Children in Hospitals" (The Charles West Lecture), *British Medical Journal,* I (1947), 125–30.

Another Englishman, James Robertson, has done us a great service in this field not only by making important observations of children in hospital and after their return home but by recording those observations in moving pictures. Some of you may have seen the film *A Two-Year-Old Goes to Hospital*[7] and its companion piece, *Mother Goes to Hospital with Child*.[8] For those of you who have not, let me briefly say that the film *A Two-Year-Old Goes to Hospital* is one of the most moving documentaries that I have ever seen. It is only partly because Laura is such an enchanting child. The film opens by showing her playing with her parents and her little friends, a perfectly healthy, well-adjusted, very mature two-and-one-half-year-old. She went into hospital, which seemed not badly run by any means, and her mother was allowed to come once a day and stay an hour. Laura had a play period with her nurse twice a day for half an hour or so. The personnel seemed kindly and warm and treated the children quite well, but in spite of this Laura got into a succession of troubles which Robertson has by now shown are quite characteristic of the responses of uprooted hospitalized young children. The first day or two she cried a great deal. This was the stage of protest. Her protest was vocal and frequent. This went on for a day and a half, perhaps two days. She then calmed down to the extent that she cried only when reminded of home or when another child nearby cried. Most of the time she just lay or sat in bed playing disinterestedly with her toys and looking utterly dejected. This stage Robertson calls "despair." She greeted her mother joyously when she came to see her, hated to see her go, and cried after she left. After another day or two—which most of us had thought of as the stage of "settling in" or, as we say in the United States, of "settling down"—the third stage occurred. Now Laura made no trouble for anyone. Everyone in the ward thought she was perfectly content. She no longer cried. She didn't even cry when her mother left. Indeed she took a long time to warm up to her mother. This behavior Robertson calls "denial." It is not indicative of settling in but of utter confusion on the part of the child. She simply cannot understand what has happened, and she appears determined to deny that it actually has happened.

After watching this child for awhile there is no wonder in your mind that when she gets home she might awake in the middle of the night, terrified that the mother who deserted her once may have deserted her again. There is no difficulty in understanding her regressions, her anger, her protests, her destructiveness. This is what I meant when I said that we have to put ourselves into

[7] J. Robertson, *A Two-Year-Old Goes to Hospital* (film), Tavistock Clinic, England.
[8] J. Robertson, *Mother Goes to Hospital with Child* (film), Tavistock Clinic, England.

another's skin. We must at least try to feel how Laura felt during her hospitalization. She had been with her mother hour after hour for the two and one-half
years of her life. She had had someone to turn to during even the mildest kind
of distress. Mother had been her Rock of Gibraltar, and suddenly the unbeliev-
able happened: the rock crumbled and disappeared. I do not think it is over-
sentimentalizing to say that the apparent desertion of this loved, needed person is
a catastrophe that a two-and-one-half-year-old just cannot understand.

Mother Goes to Hospital with Child is a marvelous contrast. Sally is not as
engaging a child as Laura, but she is very attractive. Mother goes into hospital
with her and takes her immediately to her little cubicle, which contains only a
crib for Sally, a cot for Mother, a chair and wash basin. The difference from
Laura's hospitalization is that mother does everything for Sally just as she has
always done at home. If it were not for the fact that doctors come in and hurt
her so often she might think she were on a holiday. Mother bathes her and
dresses her, feeds her, and sits by her bed when she is falling asleep at night and
is by her side when she wakes up in the morning. Sally has no feeling of having
been deserted. Therefore, she develops no protests. There is no need for depression or denial. When she returns home she is not ripe soil for the development
of posthospital emotional disturbances.

There have been other trials like this—some in our country. A few have been
described in the literature. One took place in Flemington, New Jersey, in the
Hunterton Hospital, and was reported by Dr. Trussel and Mr. Hunt,[9] chief
pediatrician and administrator, respectively. They conclude that this form of
pediatric visiting has been "uniformly and gratifyingly favorable." Follow-up
visits on discharged children reveal "a striking absence of phobic or other behav-
iorial disturbance." Unfortunately, this study was not quantitative. Since it was
not controlled we do not know how many children had phobic disturbances
before the system was initiated or what has happened since.

Our own experience here at the Children's Medical Center has been limited.
In the main it has been highly successful. I am so well satisfied with the way
living in has worked out at the Johns Hopkins that the new Greater Baltimore
Medical Center pediatric department has been set up to accommodate the maximum possible number of mothers. Most of the pediatric area has been divided
into two-bed rooms that can accommodate two children or a mother and her child.
If enough mothers want to stay we are willing to cut our income down by an

[9] A. D. Hunt, Jr., and R. E. Trussel, "They Let Parents Help in Child Care," *Modern Hospital*, LXXXV (1955), 89–91.

appreciable amount, because we are all agreed that this is the ideal way to handle sick children.

So far we have talked only about the child. Living in also presents advantages to the mother. When we do not permit the mother to come into the hospital with her child we are really saying, "You have done a fine job with your child when she was well. You have done a good job when she was moderately sick. But now that she is very sick she does not need you anymore." What we really mean is, "You will clutter up the ward; you will make it untidy; you will take up the house officers' time; you will ask too many questions; you will get in the way of the terribly busy nurses; you will see too many of the mistakes that we make. Finally, you will take up space which could be occupied by a $30-a-day patient!" A sensible, strong, self-reliant mother will recognize the first statement as foolish and may not pay too much attention to it. A weaker, a less secure mother may be further weakened if she really believes that she will be of no help to her very sick child. She will be confirmed in her own inadequacy, and we will have lost a great opportunity to let her gain self-assurance by allowing her to take an active part in the treatment of her child. Furthermore, from the point of view of surgeons and physicians who must anticipate aftercare in the case of a prolonged convalescence or a long disease the mother can learn a great deal in the hospital. She can be taught to dress wounds, to care for a colostomy, to prepare a difficult diet, and so on. She can learn from the experts in our Child Life Program how to handle a child physically and psychologically throughout a long illness.

The mother who has been denied the invaluable experience of being in the hospital with her child during the acute phase of her illness will almost certainly be less able to cope with the emotional disturbances that may appear when the child returns home. Her bonds with the child would have been strengthened by being present in the hospital, by observing the evidence of her child's real need for her.

In addition, there are other mothers in the hospital with their own sick children. Thus each mother does not feel that she is unique, singled out by a malign fate to have a sick child. There are mothers there who have children sicker than hers. These mothers support one another, cheer one another, give one another self-confidence.

There are also advantages to residents and nurses. The resident and the nurse are too prone to treat the child as the isolated individual he is not. He and she are too slow to learn about the child's position within his familial environment, his other associations and attachments, and how these are handled by his mother and father. If parents are not present they have to learn this secondhand. The resident and nurse can learn many of these things if the mother lives in and the father comes in periodically. They may make some shocking discoveries indeed when they watch Mother with her child from morning to night. They can be of tremendous help on ward rounds when they tell us observations of this nature as well as about the child's appetite, elimination, and the results of calcium, phosphorous, and catecholamine excretion tests.

There are disadvantages, too, to the hospital. Mothers take up valuable space for which the hospital is usually not recompensed adequately. They also make the job of keeping the hospital tidy a little more difficult. Mothers see mistakes and they are not loathe to comment upon them. They ask innumerable questions and they compare answers given by different members of the medical hierarchy. This does not mean that they should not be permitted to ask questions. Instead we should be more careful to give them correct answers.

Mothers are very cheap help and very good help. They can do all those things which a nurse's aide would have to do—and do them better. A lot of them like to visit with children whose mothers are not able to be present. They help the hospital's image within the community. Teaching hospitals in particular have long been thought of as cold places where one experiments upon the children who are admitted. It is tremendously valuable to us to bring mothers in and let them see that we are indeed warmly and deeply interested in their children and in them. In the unhappy situation in which the medical profession finds itself today vis-à-vis the public, the images of both doctors and hospitals could stand a little polishing and refurbishing.

The basic question then is, "Is the price of separation too high?" Is 14 out of 100 severely disturbed children in the over-all and 7 out of 100 severely disturbed for at least 3 months after hospitalization too high a price to pay for not letting mother live in? For three-year-olds and younger, is it realistic to protect half of them from serious personality changes, many of which persist? To me it is. If administrators or residents or nurses object, let them look at what every surgeon has to do when he operates. Operating room techniques must be carried out without omitting one single ritualistic detail. This is time-consuming and expensive, but do we ever think for a moment of omitting a procedure that prevents wound infections? Why then should we think for a moment that it is not equally mandatory to do those things we have to do to prevent emotional and even intellectual damage, even though they, too, may be cumbersome and expensive?

I should like to end with a question taken from Matthew's report of the Sermon on the Mount. It reads, "Or what man among you, whom if his son ask bread, will he give him a stone?"

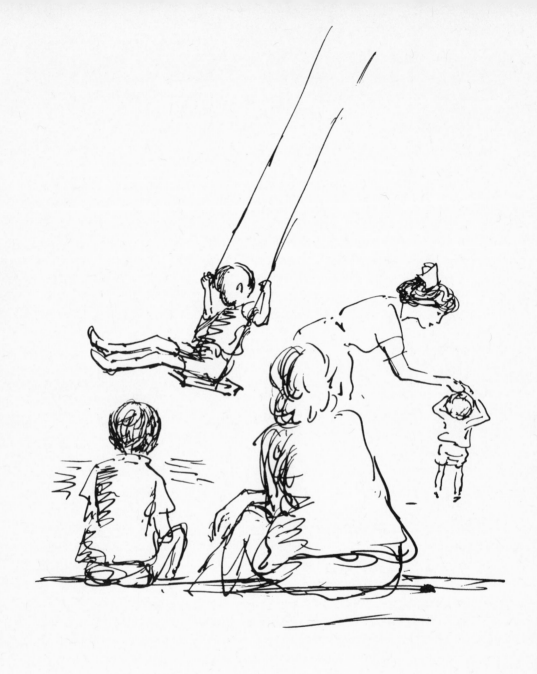

Chapter IV

THE IMPORTANCE OF PLAY FOR THE CHILD IN THE HOSPITAL

Paul Lemkau, M.D.*

One must stress the importance of play in a child's life. Play is not for the most part a matter of planned activity. When a child is in his natural habitat—if the environment is ever natural in a civilized culture—there is an internal developmental force that makes him want to exercise emerging functions. He is not content to have the ability to do something without utilizing it. Furthermore, the child wants to try what is just beyond his capacities.

Those who have watched a three-year-old struggling to ride a tricycle have seen that the alternation of flexion and extension of the legs becomes confusing at times; the tricycle won't go where the child wants it to. In this situation the child may become so frustrated that he kicks the tricycle as though it were alive, as though it had a mind of its own. He expects to be able to do something that is just over the border of possibility at the moment.

There is a kind of inevitability about the maturation of the muscular system and particularly the nervous system. There is an inevitable succession of abilities that emerge—sitting up, crawling, standing, walking—progressions of development that take place almost entirely because of internal maturational forces—if the environment is a normal one.

The chronological emergence of these events varies quite markedly from child

* Professor of Mental Hygiene, School of Hygiene and Public Health.

to child. Gesell became interested in the question of whether one could train a child to walk more quickly than it otherwise would, and he set up an experiment with a pair of identical twins to test this possibility. He tried very hard to teach one to walk, while the other he allowed to go along without any special training in this regard. He found they both walked about the same time. The nervous system seemed to be responding at its own rate rather than at an induced rate.

The folklore passed down from family to family, from generation to generation, takes these facts into consideration, and if one observes families carefully one can see the pattern of folklore stimuli that enter a child's life. Nobody thinks about these things very much because they are so ingrained in our culture. They are so much a part of that entity that is often called "mother instinct" or "parent instinct" (which on examination turns out to be largely a series of learned patterns) that we don't often bother to determine how they got there and what they are for. Yet entertainment for children incorporates folklore patterns quite clearly. One of the earliest, the patty-cake exercise, is part of the development of bilateral flexion. The infant cannot separate his two hands to deal with two separate things, but he can very well bring them together to patty-cake. Furthermore, he gets satisfaction out of this exercise. A little later we play peekaboo with the child. This very interesting game probably has something to do with the state of consciousness of the child and the condition of his memory. When the child can't see you, he probably really thinks you are gone. The event of your return when he takes his hands off his eyes or you take your hands off your eyes is an enormous event that is much more important for him than for us. In teaching peekaboo, folklore teaches the realization that things are there even though you can't see them.

Most families who have an unmarried uncle are very much aware of what can happen when, sharing the pride of the father, he picks up the six-month-old baby and, instead of cuddling it, tosses it in the air. The baby cries. As soon as the Moro reflex (a very interesting reflex in which the infant, deprived of support or hearing certain rasping sounds, jumps and cries) disappears, between six and nine months, the baby enjoys the tossing games very much. The inexperienced uncle doesn't know enough to check to see whether the Moro reflex is absent. Because he isn't used to listening to the baby's language of the cry and the jerk, he doesn't realize that this isn't a happy game for the child.

Thus the satisfactions of exercising a new function are built into folklore. It is quite clear that the enjoyment depends not only on the adults in the environment but also on the exercises themselves.

The balking of function is likely to interfere with its development. Interference is directly related to how rapidly the function would normally have developed. Swaddling, for example, has been criticized very strongly in modern times because, if continued too long, it blocks movement. On the other hand, some have pointed out that swaddling can reduce the shock of coming into a free environment after the long confinement in the uterus. Swaddling denies the child the satisfaction and the stimulus for the next move, for the emergence of the next set of reflexes that can give him further satisfaction.

The subject of the reduction of stimuli was first introduced into the American literature by Chapin in the early 1900s.[1] He was able to show that an unstimulated child would develop what was then called "marasmus." Such infants present a wizened little-old-man appearance, with a pot belly and very thin extremities. They whimper instead of crying, have chronic diarrhea, and shortly develop a low hemoglobin. If left in the unstimulated condition, the process will proceed to death. Chapin showed that the discharge of such children from the hospital brought a very rapid restoration of vigorous health; if they remained in the hospital conditions that prevailed at the turn of the century, they tended to die. What the child encountered was a kind of blank wall instead of a stimulating group of people around him. This very obviously interrupted development and interrupted it very seriously.

The emotional shock of hospitalization can block intake from the environment. A child preoccupied with his internal feelings is to some extent blinded to what goes on around him. One of the reasons one tries to prepare a child for hospitalization is to see to it that the emotional shock of the changed situation will not narrow his perceptive sphere to such an extent that he will not be able to receive stimuli from the environment. Spitz[2] has demonstrated these situations in excellent films. He implies that this reaction of narrowed perception in the child is related to a kind of depressive mood that blocks reception of stimuli from the environment.

It is an old cliché but nevertheless a true one that the child's work in this world is to play. The child's service to society is to develop, and one of the principle tasks of development is to play, to move, to do things, and to respond to stimuli. It is generally recognized that at least in the earlier years of a child's existence, the stimuli for this kind of activity have to be rather general and, for

[1] H. D. Chapin, "A Plan of Dealing with Atrophic Infants and Children," *Archives of Pediatrics*, XXV (1908), 491–96.

[2] R. H. Spitz, *Grief* (film). Available through New York University Film Board, New York.

the most part, unplanned. There is an enormous amount of it in nursery rhymes, in the games that I have mentioned, and in many others that society has ready for the child when he is developed enough to receive them. However, planning and activity in the preschool period are now considered so important for children denied general stimuli by reason of their parents' poverty in pocketbook, ideas, or both that special programs have been created to furnish them on a massive scale.

A new translation of the German text, *Cerebral Function in Infancy and Childhood,* by Peiper,[3] draws together some of the material indicating why this issue of early stimulation demands our concern.

In times past, damages caused by institutionalization have cost the lives of many infants. Particularly notorious were the foundling homes, which offered mothers an opportunity to get rid of their illegitimate and even their legitimate children through the turnstile box without being identified. But despite all good intentions, the separation of mother and child usually caused the death of the children. [Peiper, 1958 (117)]

For a long time, the task of raising infants in institutions could not be accomplished at all satisfactorily, since the mortality of the children admitted was alarmingly high. In 1858, the State Foundling Home in Prague thus had a mortality rate of 103.1%.

This is like the success rate of an obstetrical service that runs to 197 per cent. One patient is admitted and two are discharged, but here the discharge rate by death was 103 per cent of the admissions.

This figure is explained by the fact that not only all 2,831 newly admitted children died, but also those surviving from the previous year. (STEINERT, 1921). According to the statistics of the Charité-Annals [17, 106 (1892)], 174 of 176 children suffering from diseases classified as "atrophia infantum" or a "debilitas vitae" [tabes mesenterica] died in HENOCH's Berlin University Pediatric Clinic in the fiscal year 1890 to 1891. The two remaining children by no means recovered, but were reported as still in the hospital at the end of the fiscal year. FINKELSTEIN (1938) saw 70% of the infants admitted die in the same clinic, then under HEUBNER, in the year 1894–1895. He was able to save the remaining infants from death only by returning them to their families as quickly as possible. In 1898 he was still of the opinion that the mortality in pediatric hospitals under the best conditions could fall below 40%, but his low figure would be exceptional.

In 1909, SCHELBLE reported on an institutional mortality of 90% in originally healthy infants who were institutionalized only for shelter. When these infants were placed individually in homes with ordinary foster mothers, only 10 to 15% of them died. From 1903 to 1906, SCHLOSSMANN (1913, 1920) observed a mortality of 71.5% in 165 infants in a children's home, i.e., in really healthy infants, although the home was kept clean and the nurses had a great sense of responsibility. After a thorough reform in infant care, the mortality fell to 16.8% from 1907 to 1912.

The cause of death in these infants was not only the kind of deprivation of

---

[3] Albrecht Peiper, *Cerebral Function in Infancy and Childhood* (New York: Consultants Bureau, 1963).

stimuli with which we are concerned today. It also included all the factors of uncontrolled contagion and infection that were rampant in those days. But the fact remains that such terms as "atrophia infantum" imply a lack of growth, and it is obvious also that these infants were deprived of some of their protective devices, their protective physiologic functions, in this setting. Another quote from this book is particularly interesting.

That even the young child needs stimulation is evident in a fairy tale reported in the chronicle of SALIMBENE VON PARMA (thirteenth century): Emperor Frederick II wished to find out what language types and patterns boys would have after growing up, if they had never before talked to anybody. He therefore told the wet nurses and nurses to feed, bathe, and clean the children, but otherwise pay them no attention or speak to them. He wished to determine whether they would speak Hebrew, the oldest language, or Greek, Latin, Arabic, or perhaps the language of their parents. His efforts were in vain, since all the boys died, "for they could not live without the clapping of hands and the cheerful faces of their wet nurses."

Lack of stimulation has an even greater effect in young children after infancy. At home there is always something going on and life is never so dull and monotonous as it is in an institution. Parents, siblings, other relatives, and visitors bring more than enough entertainment and do not let boredom develop. Outings mean new and joyfully welcomed events, natural for the adult, but for the child, experiences in a never dreamed of colorful world. A dog is really an experience for him; he sees it, strokes it, hears it bark, and becomes frightened and fearful of it. However, the child in an institution knows a dog only from pictures or as a toy. He spends his life in an unchanging environment which, with its regular schedule and continuously repeated daily routine, offers nothing new to him. The furniture in the room may be the most practical, but the room lacks the many objects which a room at home contains, and in its bare plainness it is sometimes more reminiscent of a prison than of a nursery.

Most of us have never known the horrors of the uncontrolled infectious disease period, or even the prisonlike atmosphere of early pediatric wards. But the reforms we see in operation today are based on firm ground: they are fundamental, life-saving procedures, and their absence causes not just discomfort but death—or fractional death, in terms of the interruption of the child's normal growth and development. These are not frills but essentials, and although we have progressed far beyond the period when death was almost inevitable for an institutionalized child, we must not forget that we are dealing with life-saving measures. The sulphonimide and then the antibiotic drugs for controlling infection opened the possibility of a larger range of activity for children. With immunization and with drugs, it has been possible to allow considerable relaxation of the kind of rigid asepsis that was formerly so necessary. The mask, the white gown, the deadening, stimulus-stopping isolation, could to a large degree be forgotten when we no longer feared spreading infection. Today, when some bacteria are escaping the antibiotics and hospital cross-infections are again becoming a major problem, we must not forget that isolation and protection from infection are not the only important thing. If they again become necessary, they must be balanced by increased effort to stimulate the child.

Thus the gaiety and color that have entered the pediatric hospital—the pictures on the wall, the bright colors, the increase of stimuli for the child who is not entirely free to perceive—are not just for fun. They are for life-saving purposes. There has also been a marked increase in contact with adults while the essential medical procedures are being carried out. The child is allowed as much contact as possible with his age mates while in the hospital. Professor Harlow, at the University of Wisconsin, who has done much work on the macaques and their development, has shown that the infant monkey gains a great deal from contact with his age mates. The absence of this contact produces a very abnormal monkey, and Harlow speculates that contact with age mates may be almost as important as contact with parents or parent figures. One can observe the truth of this in the physical play of many other animals. This play is something quite essential. Children of parents with middle-class ideals but lower-class pocketbooks who grow up in neighborhoods where they are not allowed to play with "those nasty children down the street" often develop abnormal personalities. Deprived of contact with their age mates, some develop almost schizophrenic patterns.

Thus the child ought to have opportunity for physical play, even in the hospital. Not only is there need for intellectual or word contact with his fellows, but also for the physical contact that occurs when children play freely together. If this is impossible, it must be replaced as much as it can be. Playful massage is helpful, for it carries with it an emotional as well as a physical stimulus to the child's muscles.

I worked recently with a group of preschool teachers who teach cerebral palsied children. They stressed that their experience had showed that the very extensive physiotherapy on mats in the gymnasium was not enough. The children also needed contact with a hard floor, and they needed it in groups if possible. They needed the chance to shove each other around and to feel other bodies reacting to their own, even though the reaction in these children was frequently exceedingly inefficient. Thus even these severely damaged children had to have free play in order to develop satisfactorily.

There must be a wide range of objects around the child to attract his interest.

48

Although Dr. Ames of Gesell's group claims there is a clear-cut series of developmental steps, many of us think that Dr. Gesell and his group have been a bit too categorical in this, and neglectful of environmental stimuli. A variety of materials should be available to suit all ranges of interest.

The interesting object may be a pretty thing. Pretty objects teach a child that some things are valuable. These one doesn't handle. The child learns that there are different ways of appreciating things: with his eyes and with his hands. Some things he appreciates because he is able to change them, some because somebody else has made them not to be changed.

There are things that are in themselves reactive—balloons that bounce when the child touches them, dolls he can push over but that spring back with just enough resistance.

Thus there are two areas to consider—an input area we wish to enrich and an output area for expression. There is really little distinction between functions we share with most of the "lower animals" and those that are exclusively human. There is really little difference in value between the progression see, reach, grasp, and throw and the progression see, say, and sing, for example. The second progression is a distinctly human one. The first one we share with our animal forbears. The same functional analysis can be applied to both. Just as the muscles can be shown to waste in a condition of underuse or nonuse, so can these other systems be assumed to waste when not exercised, when not stimulated, when not allowed to come to executive function. Taste, see, spit, mouth—these activities are functionally analyzable in the same sphere, yet taste and see are sensory, spit and mouth have emotional overtones. We must see to it that the distinctively human emotional and intellectual functions are studied as much as the more clearly physical or "animal" ones.

We have learned that development in both spheres is of enormous concern and that failure in development means an enormous loss to society. The philosophy prevails today that even those who are not sick must have ample stimuli. This, it seems to me, is the core of the antipoverty program.

In education, the Montessori methods reveal the enormous amount of effort that goes into the planning of teaching sequences. A large amount of equipment is utilized, and a great deal of stimulus comes to the child through this elaborate teaching material.

We must, I think, pay attention to this goal of maximizing material. Cerebral palsied children have specific problems, such as a jerk that may interrupt attention to a device. Since the attention span is likely to be interrupted, not only by athetotic movements but perhaps because of other brain damage, the Montessori answer was to increase and intensify the stimulus available to the child. Administered by trained hands, such multiple stimuli should be a great boon to a child.

The aim of hospital design is to provide an environment for the child of natural, lively stimulation. If a sensory system is blocked for any reason, efforts will be made to intensify the use of others so that the total sum of stimuli will be lowered as little as possible. The hospital program should maximize the opportunity for output within the limitations imposed by the illness.

In 1951 I visited a Yugoslavian hospital for victims of bone tuberculosis. At the time, only five years after the end of World War II, bone tuberculosis was a scourge in Yugoslavia. There were hospitals all over the country for the treatment of children and adults with the disease. The hospital I saw on the Adriatic, near the city of Rijeka, was an old hotel that had been turned into a hospital by the government. In one room there were about five cribs with children ranging from two to six or eight. They had various bone lesions, most of them with hip involvement. In the same room was a woman in her thirties who was being treated for Pott's disease. We walked into the room, and I was immediately struck by the responsiveness of the children. They shouted out with great joy, and all of them responded to smiles and to speech. We were speaking English, which they didn't understand, but they responded anyway, as happy children do.

The woman was there to act as their mother. She was confined to bed, on her stomach in a full body-cast, but she was making lace. The occupational therapist was one of the cleverest I have ever met. She had tuberculosis of the hip herself—and she had taught this woman the art of lace-making of that area of Yugoslavia.

While the "mother" was making lace she was also able to keep track of the small children, to observe needs, to talk to them, and to get them to talk to each other. She was intensifying meaningful contact, so to speak. The director of this institution knew just what he was about: he wanted this woman to mother the children. She had to do so entirely with her voice. She was not just another patient. She had particular responsibilities, and these were as stimulating to her as they were stimulating and helpful to the children with her.

Much of what I have said has had to do with long-term institutionalization and hospitalization. Yet emotional shock occurs in brief hospitalization as well, although such hospitalizations present less danger of emotional omissions. By extrapolation of the findings on long-term stays, one comes to the conclusion that the best hospitalization involves the least interruption of the flow of stimuli to the child and the least interference with the flow of executive functions. We will be well advised to see to it that these factors are taken into consideration in short-term hospitalizations as well.

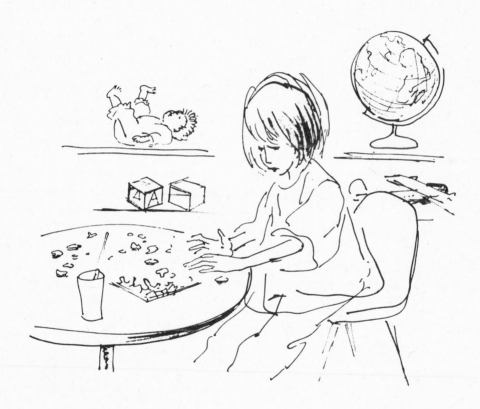

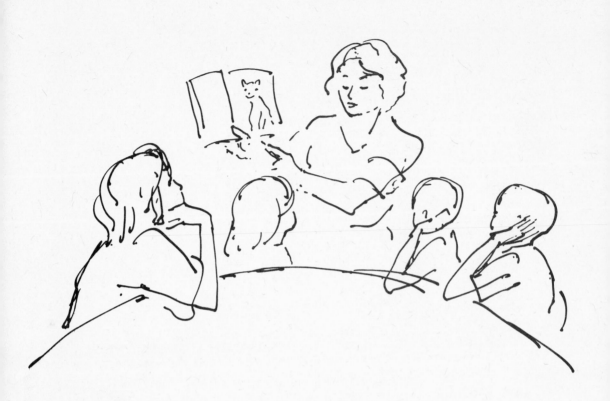

Chapter V

EDUCATIONAL NEEDS AND PROGRAMS FOR THE HOSPITALIZED CHILD

Henry M. Seidel, M.D.*

As Mammy Yokum says succinctly, "Larnin's important."

The *Maryland School Bulletin,* in an edition devoted to policies and programs for public secondary education in Maryland, puts it more sophisticatedly:

Change is an outstanding characteristic of our modern world. Power generated by hand, muscle, wind, and running water generally has been replaced by the force of machines propelled by steam, petroleum, electricity, and atomic energy. Although every generation has had to face a world different from the preceding one because of change, never before has change occurred at so fast a pace! The past fifty years have seen more changes than any previous 500 years. It is difficult to realize that in 1910 most Americans did not have electricity, telephones, and automobiles; that, before 1920, air travel and television were unknown to most people; that satellites, atomic submarines and jet-propelled airplanes are largely developments of the last ten years. As a result of the impact of technology, youth of this era will encounter rapidly rising sociological and scientific changes which their parents neither experienced nor imagined.

Demands of these changing times present a challenge of great magnitude to those engaged in education; thus, the role of education is a complex and difficult one. It must equip boys and girls to live in an increasingly intricate and demanding world and to manage constructively the social, economic, and cultural forces in that world. Moreover, in our democratic society the school has the responsibility for providing and maintaining a valid relationship between the learning experiences needed by all youth and those needed to satisfy individual interests and needs. Finally, the school has the further responsibility of providing for the development of the individual both as a human being and as a contributing member of society.[1]

* Assistant Professor of Pediatrics.
[1] Vol. XXXIX, No. 3 (April, 1963).

Mammy Yokum and the State Department of Education accentuate the premise of our discussion—that the hospitalized child does indeed have an educational need and a vital one. In my practice of pediatrics I discovered that mild short-term illness treated at home causes insistent parental pressure. Nowadays, fever occasions much less concern than missed school time. The child contributes to the pressure because of work he will miss or a test he will have to make up.

When we relate this to the hospitalized child, we must recognize additional areas. Any individual coming to the hospital brings with him his own particular personality and his own particular set of needs. Superimposed on the child's matrix of needs are three other factors. The first, of course, is the principle reason for being at the hospital: his illness. At this point, the demands of the illness are paramount. Second, when he is admitted, the child feels bewildered, victimized, and suffers hurt for being taken from his family. He views hospitalization most often as a punitive experience. Third, he brings with him the needs of the culture from which he comes and to which he will quickly return. Our children are from a world that has known no major war for twenty years, yet each has been growing in a world that has known no peace. He has also been growing in a world so well wired for communication that even the first- or second-grader is much more sophisticated, much more acutely aware of his total environment and its problems, than we were a generation or two ago. Good evidence is the impact of the death of President Kennedy on the very young and the response of many children to those four days on the television screen. Since World War II there has been a great premium on education. Perhaps the stimulus originated with *Sputnik,* but I think it would have happened anyway. Ours is a highly competitive culture. Children are tested as early as the first grade and begin to catalogue themselves into groups according to the results. Subtle, and not so subtle, competitive pressures come not only from parents fearful of their child's educational future but also from teachers and from the children themselves.

Thus the hospitalized child is a sick child, a separated child, a child in a highly competitive culture in which education often comes first. Many adults, admitted to the hospital, are excused from work, have sick leave, and are not asked to make up the time. Not so the child. When he goes back to work, to school, his largest area of experience outside home, the rest of the class has gone on its way. He must catch up and convalesce, too.

One aim of the Child Life Program in the Children's Medical and Surgical Center is to meet the psychological and the academic needs of the child. First of all, adequate outlets for rising hostility are necessary. The hospital presents a culture in microcosm which demands, for adjustment, a quick kind of social growth from the novitiate. Because of lack of experience or poor preparation, the result may be confusion. Although the doctor or the nurse may feel disposed to help the child in this direction, their primary task lies elsewhere. Inactivity of the child before a hospital television set may compound anxiety. Development may regress or be retarded.

A school program in the hospital which approximates normal educational activities can forestall this. The child can feel assured of keeping pace with his class. The hospital's concern with his education gives subtle but strong reinforcement to the feeling that he will get well.

In Chapter II Dr. J. Alex Haller, Jr., has expressed the idea that hospitalization should be a "growing adventure" for the child. An educational experience provides a familiar foothold, a means for acting out his fears, a means for providing a secure base from which to explore and profit from this new adventure. This view is supported by Hedley G. Dimock in *The Child in Hospital*. He feels the normal, everyday school experience is psychologically advantageous, that it provides a framework.

Once at "school," there are familiar paraphernalia—blackboard, chalk, erasers, the American flag, alphabet cards, textbooks, crayons, arts and crafts supplies— to counterbalance the often awesome tools of the hospital. Most important, the teacher is a familiar kind of adult, usually associated with pleasant experiences. The child thus has some idea of what is expected of him and how he will react to it. He must be helped to understand, however, that this school is only temporary.

In the hospital environment the behavior of the child is partly controlled by persons telling him to co-operate in getting well. How many thoughtless remarks have been made in this area! Given daily tests and treatments, the child may feel that any release of hostility may result either in an increase of these procedures or a failure to get well. Not expressing hostility may result in more anxiety. The school provides a setting when the child may have the opportunity to "act out" these fears without dreading medically painful or threatening consequences.

Initially the teacher may give the child this opportunity by making daily attendance, when medically possible, part of the school routine. He may be allowed to react as he sometimes does at home—by refusing to go. His mother may react in a variety of ways to this kind of reluctance, but most reactions imply that the child will ultimately attend school that day. A child may give just as many reasons for his negativism during hospitalization, but the real reason is usually a desire for attention. In releasing surface hostility, the child receives that attention. For some, this is an acceptable way of achieving positive physical contact with a mother substitute. Thus, a hand on the shoulder, a pat on the head, or a piggyback ride helps him to meet emotional needs. This, of course, is very simply a part of any healing process, the traditional "laying on of hands."

However, it should not be forgotten that some children, because of their background experience, are sincere in their negative reaction to school attendance. The child who has been labeled a "trouble maker" in school and has not fitted the popular concept of a "good pupil" may well choose the imagined fears of the hospital room rather than the real fears of the schoolroom.

Some chronically ill children undergo short-term readmissions for drug regulation and checkups. For some of these the schoolroom is the situation that produces anxiety. By learning to relate to his hospital teacher, he can eventually work himself into the schoolroom, into the development of habits and attitudes that improve social living, into the sum total of human experience.

The hospital school experience allows a continued interaction with other children, thus extending normal growth and development. The social contact that enables a youngster to make new friends, see them get well, and go home may enable him to talk about going home. The teacher at the same time provides classroom activities that reinforce or formulate a positive attitude toward school. The child is given the opportunity to achieve because he is accepted at his own academic level. For a child in the hospital, particularly one who is in for a short time only, the intrusion of hospital demands will dampen the vitality of academic performance. Thus academic demands should often be understated. Each child should be enabled also to understand his disease. When an educational goal is imposed upon a child who cannot achieve it, disappointment and increased emotional instability are to be expected. Physical and academic education should blend and be consistent with the child's handicap. With these considerations, the teacher can plan, give individual attention, and even remedy deficiencies made glaring by the large community classroom. The child can then return to school with little or no academic regression.

The teacher is not enough; the doctor and the nurse are not enough. A Child

Life Program is also needed to make the hospital experience a strengthening one by providing activities comparable to those that take place in the home and in the community outside the school. Nevertheless, the physician and the nurse are dominant figures in any hospital program. Consequently the nurse must be sensitized to all the needs of her patients. Communication with the teacher is essential to provide background for the latter on illness and readiness for the in-hospital school experience. The nurse should plan the child's daily routines to have him ready for school. Whenever possible, treatments, medications, and nursing care should revolve around the school, which can be so familiar and reassuring to the patient. Most important, perhaps, the nurse can listen with interest and communicate to the child the feeling that his efforts to meet the demands of school are worth while.

Dr. Catherine Neill, associate professor of pediatrics, extends this vital concept of co-operation and understanding to include all the hospital personnel. Thus we come to another truth—working together's important. She stresses, however, that no one who works with children who are seriously ill can ever forget that good medical and nursing care are absolutely paramount. However, there is much that a physician can contribute, even for a short-term hospitalization. The pity is that there are so few who do. Dr. Neill did a limited survey of pediatric histories. She sought to find mention of how a child was doing in school, of his level of scholastic achievement. Only one-third of the histories made any reference to the child's school situation. This is not really surprising. The principle orientation of medical education in the past has been in the direction of physical disease. Only the last fifty years have witnessed a real growth in the treatment of mental disease. Marginal problems dealing with more subtle, less life-disrupting situations have received greater attention only since World War II. The family as a unit is only recently gaining recognition. The plain fact is that most physicians leave medical school unaware and unsophisticated in the everyday problems of living—family interaction, social need, sexual orientation, the emotional response to death; however, this is changing. These problems will continue to challenge medical education.

If physicians at all levels realize and understand the educational need, they can add much to the scope and value of the child's hospitalization. Medical need is paramount. Thus the hospital team that accepts disease as an adversary and plans in terms of health must be aware that a child who sits in the hospital doing nothing depresses himself and those around him—and shares the common experience of many that hospital walls are a prison. The teacher is a bridge to the outside, and the physician must not only appreciate this fact but use it to the advantage of his patient. This makes the hospital part of the larger world and orients the child's needs to his whole environment.

The dialogue between doctor and teacher allows the child to begin to define goals that are in keeping with the limitations of his illness. For example, a child with a severe cardiac condition will no longer aspire to weight-lifting. With an awareness of his illness, he can sharpen those particular skills that can balance and refine his own self-image, his own sense of individuality. He needs to be good at something. The physician must realize his own role in providing this motivation. It is, after all, essential to therapy.

The physician, too, must reach beyond the confines of the hospital and beyond the departure of the child from the hospital. Just as the doctor is often hampered by lack of insight, so the educator, the school principal, the guidance counselor, are often handicapped by rules and regulations. In spite of the grand ideals expressed in the *Maryland School Bulletin,* too many educators think in terms of the whole student group and forget or find it impossible to adjust to the needs of the individual child. We could all profit from a little judicious rule-breaking! Certainly the physician has a heavy responsibility to seek means for increased co-operation between school and hospital personnel.

Legislative rules make it necessary to separate hospitalizations into short-term and long-term periods. The fact that the State of Maryland will begin financial support only for a child hospitalized longer than eight weeks is our point of reference. Thus a long-term hospitalization is defined as one longer than eight weeks. However, Dr. Marie Britt Rhyne, assistant professor of pediatrics at our Children's Medical and Surgical Center, has noted that as the hospital stay is lengthened, contact with home becomes dimmer and the child is faced with a greater disruption of familiar environmental and emotional ties. The need to maintain grade level is intensified. The problem is pinpointed in a magazine edited by students in Public School 354, which is maintained by the Board of Education for young tubercular patients in Baltimore City hospitals. The writer quotes the teacher: "I think the doctors and nurses believe the patients get well faster when they have regular school work to do."[2]

[2] *Hilltop News,* Tuberculosis Division of Baltimore City Hospitals, p. 17.

A good case in point is a patient of Dr. Rhyne's. A nine-year-old girl with chorea came regularly to the classroom in a wheelchair until a case of measles developed on her floor. During the two days she was kept in isolation she lost muscular control, was unable to hold a pencil, fell out of her wheelchair, and had to be fed. On returning to the classroom, there was decided improvement. She could once again stay in her chair, hold a pencil, and write her name. Diverted, she had incentive to improve and control muscle skills.

This child's story points out a dramatic change in over-all medical approach to hospitalized children—the increase in patient mobility. Children are not incarcerated in one spot any more. For example, the Children's Convalescent Hospital in Washington, D. C., has enrolled its asthmatic patients, who are frequently in the hospital for six to twelve months, in a special health school run by the D. C. Department of Education. This same hospital also has had a successful working arrangement since 1953 with a nearby public school. A representative from the hospital works with the principal and teachers in the handling of patients' behavior and medical problems.[3] This increased mobility makes a co-operative effort possible.

Unfortunately, on a country-wide basis, this kind of recognition and planning is usually deficient. In 1961, while he was a student at Antioch College, David Chandler worked in our Child Life Program for three months. He surveyed the education and recreation programs for children in two hospital groups—forty pediatric wards in general hospitals and sixty-seven children's hospitals—in the United States and Canada.

Of the forty general hospitals, slightly more than three-fourths indicated that they had a recreation program of some kind within their pediatric departments. Slightly less than three-fourths had a program of education. The extent of both types of programs varied a great deal.

The staff for education programs was most often no larger than two. Ambulant patients were taught in small classrooms. Nonambulatory patients were given tutoring at the bedside. Salaries for teachers were in almost all cases paid by the city, county, or state board of education, although a few hospitals supplemented salaries through special grants. Supplies other than textbooks were usually obtained by the hospital. Generally, educational services were offered to all chil-

[3] D. C. Widdowson, "The Hospital Teacher and the Nurse," *Nursing Outlook*, II, No. 5 (May, 1959), 273.

dren who were patients for more than ten days. Some hospitals were able to offer only tutoring.

A number of hospitals provided no educational program at all on their pediatric wards because the administration felt that the average stay was too short to make one worth while. These hospitals had, on the other hand, a greater variety of planned recreational activities than hospitals with educational programs. These activities were run by one or two persons, from the occupational therapy department, the nursing staff, volunteer groups, or from a professional department of pediatric recreation.

Salaries ranged from $3,000 to $7,800 annually for program directors. Half the hospitals had a supply budget that did not exceed $800; a few were as high as $2,000. More than one-third had no supply budget and met their needs from voluntary donations. Volunteer personnel also played a great role in supplementing the work of the full-time staff. Valuable as they were, they were often not available when needed and in addition required supervision to an extent that rendered the time investment impractical.

The sixty-seven pediatric institutions included thirty-eight general hospitals, eighteen orthopedic hospitals, and eleven chronic disease and convalescent sanatoriums. Only 22 of these had supply budgets, and these average $700; 3 hospitals exceeded $1,100. Of the 67, 4 hospitals listed the salary range for a recreation director of $3,600 to $5,500 per year. Forty-three of the hospitals had paid personnel; most had only one or two, but one had twelve. Volunteers helped out, but their numbers were not always reported. One hospital had sixty volunteers.

What is the quality and the adequacy of such programs? These are hard to measure and seem to range from very poor to very good. However, the budget figures provide a good basis for comparison. The median daily census in the pediatric institutions was seventy-three. An average annual supply budget was $700, or about $1.92 a day.

What is the quality of available education personnel? There are so few experienced hospital teachers that the competence here may be quite high. However, this quality is scattered irregularly in a very few places, and in almost all institutions the coverage is impossibly thin.

What initial steps toward improvement are in order? Improvement implies increased coverage—from a chronically deficient supply of teachers. This challenging task really does call for a special kind of teacher. She must function as a member of the hospital team, looking to the physician and nurse for briefing on the patient's physical and emotional status. Schedules must fit into the closely co-ordinated hospital program.

Flexibility in time allotments and methods is demanded by the child's changing medical condition. There is an increasing awareness of the need for special courses and other preparatory training in this field, perhaps teaching internships that provide a knowledge of basic medical mystique and a greater understanding of exceptional children.[4] The establishment of such internships would seem a practical recognition of the unique contribution of the hospital teacher to the care and encouragement of the sick child and would do much to insure mutual understanding and teamwork. It would also provide greater opportunity for research and expansion of supportive and rehabilitative programs in this relatively new and challenging field of teaching the hospitalized child. And, most important, it may begin to attract the kind of teacher needed, one who has (1) ability to deal with a variety of children at different grade levels, with different backgrounds, and of many ages; (2) skill in methods and a strong background in subject matter; (3) a wide repertoire of experience in home, playground, schoolroom, and summer camp; (4) enough perception and flexibility to understand quickly each child's emotional and educational needs; (5) willingness to work irregular, long hours; (6) tolerance of interruptions in routine, frequent manifestations of behavioral extremes, and frustration; and (7) capacity to deal objectively with pain and death. Perhaps such a paragon can be described as a physically and emotionally healthy man or woman who can see that a day spent teaching a child who may die tomorrow has merit among the achievements of men. Fortunately, there are such people.

It is also necessary to view the problems of the community beyond hospital walls, which brings us to yet another truth: Money's important. For more than ten years I have watched with interest the efforts of parents' and teachers' groups to manipulate the budget allotments for education in the city, the county, and the state. Legislators, beset by pressures from multiple sources and wary of the taxpayer's eye, constitute a constricting counterbalance.

Thus it is important to ask: Who is going to pay for our proposals? How can the supply budgets be increased? Who will pay salaries, and if the city or the

4 *Ibid.*

state pays them, will they allow the teacher to function independently of the system? If the answer to the last question is "No," can outside control be congruous with the paramount demands of hospital care? Can an adequate system of communications be readily maintained in an ongoing arrangement? On a country-wide basis, can the diverse approaches of countless communities find rapport with the relatively consistent patterns of hospital care? And, finally, what of a hospital such as ours with admissions from everywhere? Which community becomes responsible for which child and under what terms? Would the child from Passaic, New Jersey, be neglected because his hometown refused support or because the line of communication functioned too slowly? It is worth pointing out that in a recent tally, admissions at the Children's Medical and Surgical Center comprised the following: 61 per cent from Baltimore City, 1 per cent from Baltimore County, and 38 per cent from the rest of Maryland, the United States, and elsewhere.

Partial answers to some of these questions can be had from people in the hierarchy of the state and city Departments of Education. I found them interested and willing to talk, but affected by needs other than mine.

It was, first of all, pointed out that our community does accept responsibility for children hospitalized, or out of school for medical reasons, for eight weeks or longer. There is at the present time no prospect for including children in the hospital for shorter periods. In addition, if there is state or city financial support, education supervision of the hospital teacher becomes necessary. The problem is to blend this kind of supervision with medical demands.

I heard such discouraging statements on education in the hospital as, "A high percentage of short-term hospitalized children don't need it"—and yet, in our terms, they most certainly do—or, "By the time we found out what the individual child needs, he'd be back to school. All the rules and regulations handicap quick decisions as to needs." However, even now, there are children participating from their homes in their own classroom's work on a state-wide telephone hookup. It utilizes a speaker in the home and in the class, as well as telephone relays. The child participates directly and actively. The budget confines the current program, of course, but ultimately hospitals, too, will be similarly wired.

From officials at the city level, I learned that because the state underwrites a large portion of the special education budget, state policy dictates city practice. It is because of this kind of pragmatism that I believe all citizens should be vigorous letter-writers—to city councilmen and state legislators.

Dr. Harrie Selznik, who oversees the management of special educational problems in Baltimore City, says that this area foresees no change in the near future.
There are obvious budget limitations. Communications and continuity are significant problems. There is a need for a working relationship with the teacher.
To make it meaningful takes time and communications involving the physician,
paramedical hospital staff, and the teacher. The clerical responsibility alone is
imposing. Because these issues are not easily resolved, the experience for the
short-term hospitalized patient would turn out to be more recreational than
educational. How is the teacher to identify need, provide thoughtful organization, a good lesson plan, and continuity with the school before and after hospitalization? Dr. Selznik pointed out, "Education should have continuity, and I
have difficulty seeing it as part of an ongoing program of education. At this point,
I am hard put to justify this utilization when there are children who have
extended need draining our present personnel."

Dr. Selznik said further that even if the hospital trained and provided its own
teacher, he could not provide funds for salary. However, he was aware of the
need and would be willing, when possible, to provide books and visual aids.

He cited his co-operation with Mrs. Peggy Cluster at the "short-term school"
in the University of Maryland Hospital. Mrs. Cluster has been at the University
Hospital for four of the program's nine or ten years and is sensitive to all the
factors involved. She feels that the great many culturally deprived children in
her hospital could benefit tremendously from planned knowledge and stimulation
through new experiences. "Ideally," she commented, "the schoolroom should be
large enough so that all school-age children are included in activities, bed
patients as well as wheelchair and ambulatory ones. But if this is not possible,
then the program can be worked out to take care of most of the wheelchair and
ambulatory children in the morning, and in the afternoon the teacher can spend
some time at the bedside with the other children. Thought must be given to
include the bed-rest children in the total planning so that they, too, feel a part
of the schoolroom though separated physically in the mornings. . . . The actual
plans for the work and play to be carried on in the schoolroom on any given
day depend entirely on which individual children will be present on that particular day. The atmosphere and the planning necessarily must be fluid and
relaxed—the basic axiom is the individual child and how we can help him on
that day."

Mrs. Cluster provides for me the balance between the obvious needs of the child and the obvious problems of the community as forthrightly declared by Dr. Selznik. We know that the long-term hospitalized child's educational needs have already been accepted as a community responsibility in most areas. We wish to see this extended to include the short-term hospitalized child. We can best do this by simply beginning, as we have, to satisfy this need from within the hospital. A successful and growing program, supported actively by all of us in the hospital environment, can generate a community awareness that may spread even to those who provide funds.

For the present, responsibility for the short-term hospitalized child will rest with the hospital. We began viewing this problem from the point of view of the child committed to education. We continued with the point of view of the school pressed to educate in a rapidly exploding, moving population with changing social values, pressed to decide whether every child, in the full sense of the American dream, shall get his education.

We must conclude that for every hospitalized child the step toward providing a continuing flow of education is a logical one, a sound one. But, faced by present needs and restricted funds, this step should provide just that—a flow and not a torrent. A flow implies a nonpressurized approach, free of the pseudocultural educational vise that our society seems to be constantly tightening. This latter includes a misdirected, vicarious education, which is learning by an individual— a child—to gratify the emotional need of his parents.

One may question if extending education through the time a child has appendicitis isn't really carrying things too far. I don't believe it is. We all need a continuing sense of achievement, and if, for any disruptive reason, we are removed from our normal milieu, we need the assurance that we can return to that environment unhindered. If there must be hindrance, a background of support and encouragement is vital.

Let me repeat: my concept of the educational need of the hospitalized child implies a flow and not a torrent—a part of the supportive environment which speeds recovery and return to the realistic goals of achievement. This calls for a perspective that defines education as a tool, in the hospital and in life itself. I would like to have it stand apart from the corrupted view of educational need— the torrent—that so seriously and adversely influences so many children today.

While our means for implementing these programs grow, the greatest stimulus should come from the hospital, where the medical need comes first and where the flow can be controlled. Ultimately, the entire community will participate. Then, we will hopefully have learned to foster the development of each child with the right admixture of medicine, play, and school.

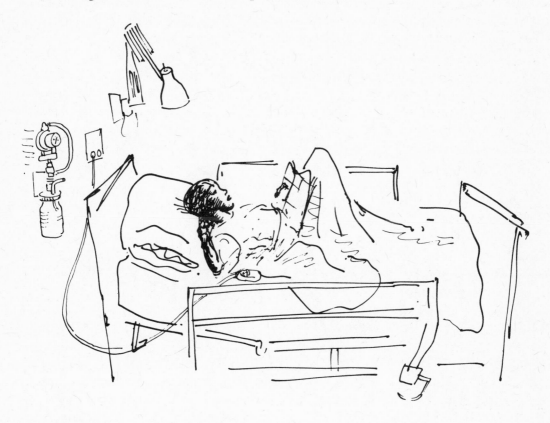

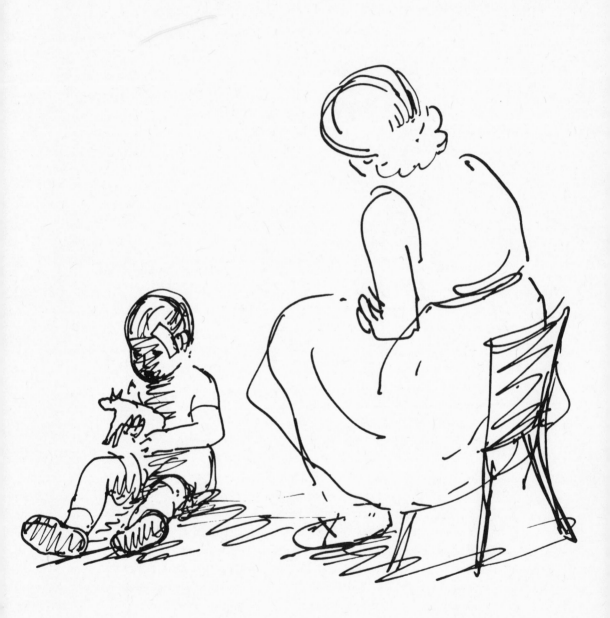

Chapter VI

THE CHILD AND HIS FAMILY AT HOME AFTER HOSPITALIZATION

*Catherine A. Neill, M.D.**

Once the child is safely home with his family after hospitalization, the major objectives of inpatient care have been achieved. Nevertheless, his readjustment to life at home, if indeed a readjustment is needed, involves points on which information is still spotty, subjective, and more inadequate than we might wish.

Anyone who remembers a personal experience with hospitalization as a child is impressed by the major role of the parents both before and after hospitalization. It is difficult to talk about the significance of parents without sounding a little platitudinous, but the fact remains that the individual child is a star in a constellation, the constellation being his family. As Dr. Schaffer emphasized in Chapter III, not the least advantage of a living-in program or of the extensive visiting periods that are now customary in most children's hospitals is that the doctors and nurses are continually forced, sometimes even against their will, to remember the child in the context of his family rather than to think of him in isolation. On the whole, the child who has been well handled in the hospital and returns home in good physical health will adjust very rapidly to the outside world if his home is a happy one and he feels the security of being loved.

Once the child is home we must think of him as an outpatient. Clearly he has, and always had, many identities other than patient, such as son, nephew,

* Associate Professor of Pediatrics.

brother, grandson, pupil, or boy next door. Now he has lost one identity, that of an inpatient, and if he is fortunate may never resume it until late in adult life. Many studies have been conducted on children as inpatients, and a few have borne invaluable fruit. Outpatient pediatric medicine, or follow-up care, in all its aspects has been studied less well and is undoubtedly less highly regarded.

The results of this comparative neglect are readily apparent by simple inspection of a modern institution such as our own Children's Medical and Surgical Center. The inpatient areas, in addition to their pleasant appearance, contain at least a hundred new ideas and improvements in architectural design. The whole outpatient area, brightly colored though it is, contains in my view only one new idea, the carrousel! Yet the material for long-term studies, follow-up, natural history studies, and good care for relatively minor ailments lies in this outpatient area of medicine.

The major factors that influence the child after he has returned home are clearly the medical state of his health and the nature of his home, both on a psychological and a more material level. In the great majority of cases, fortunately, the medical state of the child is excellent. For example, if he leaves the hospital after a tonsil or hernia operation, one postoperative visit is usually sufficient. The child can then go about his normal life with very little reminder of his hospitalization. At the other extreme, the child with leukemia must return regularly, have many studies, much medication, often many hospitalizations, and will usually die within a few years. Intermediate is the child with heart disease, in whom prolonged convalescence is needed but who, in many instances, will ultimately be able to lead a normal life.

A particularly difficult group to handle, and one to which a great deal of care and attention has been devoted, includes children with rheumatic fever. A child going home after an episode of this illness needs close follow-up and treatment for any fresh streptococcal infection that may arise. Yet many of these children have been left with no heart disease and therefore should not be at all restricted. It does not take a great deal of imagination to realize that unless extreme care is exercised by all concerned, the rather difficult concept that this is a normal child, yet one for whom there is particular anxiety about recurrent streptococcal infections, may be misinterpreted by even the most intelligent and co-operative parents. In spite of repeated reassurances, these parents may naturally feel that a child who needs careful follow-up must have something wrong with him and, therefore, should be restricted in playing games and other activities. At the other extreme, there is the danger they may feel that the child has nothing wrong with him and that there is no need to take his sore throats particularly seriously. These contrasting groups naturally require different methods of handling, different methods of administration of their outpatient visits—altogether a good deal more imaginative adaptation than we have yet developed. Some of the organizational and staff morale aspects of prolonged follow-up in rheumatic patients are interestingly discussed by Feinstein *et al.*[1]

In order to consider this subject in a relatively logical sequence, I have arbitrarily divided children leaving the hospital into five groups and have confined my attention to two aspects: the major role of the hospital in each group at the time of the child's discharge and the areas in which improvement seems to be needed.

In the first group, Group A, is a child who has had a satisfactory hospital experience, with a relatively brief hospitalization, and a mother who has either lived in or been a frequent visitor. The medical and nursing staff have been kind, patient, and gentle, and the Child Life Program has been an active part of his stay. He is about to go back to a good home with balanced parents who have, between them, relatively few "complexes" and psychological difficulties. Such parents should be given clear-cut, simple, follow-up instructions on how long he should be allowed up each day, diet, medications, and, of course, an appointment for specific follow-up visits. At the time of discharge the family doctor must be fully informed of all follow-up wishes.

In summary, then, the role of the hospital is to pass a child back as rapidly, as pleasantly, and as cheerfully as possible to his normal environment and *to relinquish hold*. (See Table VI-1.)

TABLE VI-1

GROUP A: BENIGN HOSPITALIZATION AND GOOD HOME

I. Clear-cut, simple follow-up instructions
    A. Length of ambulatory activity
    B. Diet
    C. Medications, removal stitches, etc.
II. Family doctor fully informed
III. Pass the child back to his normal environment
IV. Relinquish hold

[1] A. R. Feinstein *et al.*, "Rheumatic Fever in Children and Adolescents," *Annals of Internal Medicine,* IX, Suppl. 5 (1964).

This does not mean that *no* follow-up visits should be scheduled, but it does imply that visits should be limited in number and treatment simple in scope. This is all very logical, but in practice amazing problems may develop. Sometimes there are repeated phone calls back and forth about the patient. The mother may wish to bring him in to be seen more times than is medically necessary, or there may be prolonged and sometimes acrimonious correspondence regarding insurance and other reports. These problems are fortunately rare when there is a good home and where the administrative arrangements are of high caliber.

In the second group of patients, Group B, the child has had a bad hospital experience for some reason, because of a long admission, multiple painful procedures, friction between parents and hospital staff, or some other distressing causes—which, unfortunately, may include bad management. The child is returning to a reasonably good home, recovered from his illness. Detailed follow-up instructions are important. In view of the stress to which the family has been subjected, it is ideal if these instructions can be given with *both* parents present. The family doctor should be fully informed and specifically warned of any complications that may arise. It is useful for him to know that the child may demonstrate various psychological reactions after his hospitalization: nightmares, bed-wetting, temper tantrums, and so forth.

I think I differ from some physicians, and certainly from many nurses, in believing that it is not very helpful to the parents to discuss these reactions in great detail. I do not think, for example, that it is helpful to a mother who has had her child in the hospital for several months, some of that time on the critical list, to be told that the child may have nightmares for a few months.

This is a debatable area, and I vary my tactics according to the type of mother with whom I am dealing. Many parents today are very well informed on these psychological aspects, and if they ask questions they should be honestly answered to the best of one's ability. Indeed, if he is sufficiently receptive the physician continues to learn a great deal of new information from patients and their parents. More important than discussing details of things that could conceivably go wrong is to convey two major ideas to the parents. First, you are returning to them a child who has been extremely ill, but who is now better and who will ultimately return to normal. In so doing you express your confidence in their ability to handle this child. Dr. Schaffer alluded to this as an instillation of confidence in the mother's ability to take care of her child. This instillation of intelligent confidence is most important. The whole process is greatly helped, particularly if the patient is a sick infant, if the mother comes in for a few days prior to discharge and does practically all the handling of the infant during that time.

Hospital personnel often forget to verbalize the mutual feeling that the long, difficult hospitalization has indeed been an ordeal for the parents as well as for the patient. The concept of commiseration is rather unfashionable, for we all like to believe that we are well and strong and can live cheerfully and bravely through all misfortunes. It therefore becomes difficult to commiserate with parents without appearing to be patronizing. On the other hand, some of the problems in the postdischarge or posthospitalization period may arise from the fact that the mother and father have actually had an exceedingly rough time during their child's illness. The child has had cards, flowers, and continuous sympathy and has possibly become thoroughly spoiled. The mother, on the other hand, is completely exhausted, and nobody seems to have the slightest sympathy for her or to show signs of realizing that she has been through any kind of ordeal. It is sometimes helpful to warn the mother that she may go through a period of feeling tired and unhappy herself.

If the illness has been serious and long, the other children in the family will have been neglected. Thus they have a grievance, whether they verbalize it or not, and they will often be very difficult. Although they will not usually express this grievance by being unkind to the sick child who has come home from the hospital, they may do so in many other ways. An interesting example of this occurred recently in a very fine family with an excellent home. A number of family tensions were only dimly recognized when the patient came in. Thought to have rheumatic fever, she had been in bed for three months, the center of attention. Meanwhile her sixteen-year-old sister left home with a highly unsatisfactory young man whom she ultimately did not marry. This episode can not be attributed entirely to the sister's desire to refocus some of the limelight on herself, but there is very little doubt that this factor played a role.

Group B children need careful follow-up. It is important to make these follow-up visits brief, pleasant, and as infrequent as possible. Thus when the child comes to the hospital everything should be organized so that the necessary tests will be performed in the minimum of time, neither preceded by a long wait nor accompanied by many needles. Some of these very traumatic hospitalizations can have the edge removed over subsequent months of follow-up as the child comes back to the hospital, and, if possible, sees the same physician repeatedly under pleasant and nonpainful circumstances. (See Table VI-2.)

Group C children are becoming more and more frequent problems. These are

TABLE VI-2

GROUP B: BAD HOSPITAL EXPERIENCE, GOOD HOME, RECOVERED

I.   Detailed follow-up instructions for both parents

II. Family doctor fully informed

III. Follow-up visits brief, pleasant, infrequent

IV. Relinquish hold

V.   Sympathetic reassurance of parents by hospital staff

children with benign hospitalizations who go back to homes that are either emotionally or economically poor. I frankly do not know how to handle the emotionally deprived group. With the tremendous social pressures to marry and have children, a woman may have children when she is not really very maternal. She may have been an excellent executive secretary and would have made a very fine spinster aunt. Since the role of the spinster aunt is no longer a popular one in our society, she has married and has a child of whom she is not really very fond. Thus she may have brought the child to the hospital not for medical advice but because she wanted him changed. After she has him home for a week or so she realizes that he is still the same little Willie, the same ordinary cantankerous little fellow who is neither as tall as the boy next door nor as bright as his cousin, but now is minus his tonsils. He still is not perfect and looks no more like a future president of the United States than when he went into the hospital. This situation is not really very rare, particularly if something major such as heart surgery has been undertaken during the hospitalization. Such mothers are not talked about a great deal. I certainly do not know how to handle them, and I don't believe the hospital has a plan for handling them. Unless some very major family stress is revealed, I personally think it is probably best for the hospital not to interfere but instead to allow the family doctor to take over and indeed to request him to do so.

It is quite important for us to realize that not every child who goes back to a nice clean, tidy home is necessarily going back to a good home. If the home is a scene of strife, the mother will at some point realize this is bad for the child and will reach out for help. Probably the role of the hospital is to be available, non-critical, warm, and sympathetic.

The economically poor home is, of course, a commonplace. The child from such a home should be recognized when he is admitted and the nature and scope of the problem worked out by the hospital staff. The key figure in this therapy is the social worker. In helping to plan the follow-up care of such a child, we should use the available social agencies: public health nurses and welfare aid if indicated—without overlap by the various agencies.

In a home both emotionally and economically unsatisfactory, the mother is very often not the central figure. Now that the existence of poverty in this country is finally officially recognized, there is discussion of the breakdown of family life. This may well be a misnomer, because there may have been no real family life. Among the Hopkins clientele this particular family group is at present predominantly, but by no means entirely, Negro.

The responsible figure in this society is very often the grandmother. The children from these homes are cared for not by the mother but by the grandmother, who also looks after one or two young children of her own and, possibly, neighbor's children as well. She is usually a sensible person who has acquired a wide basic experience in pediatrics. I believe the hospital should work with this responsible figure *and* with the mother in order to protect any potential mother-child relationship.

For Group C, follow-up should be performed by the family physician. A similar disposition is often suggested for the children going back to an economically poor home. This solution is particularly popular with hospital administrators of large institutions whose outpatients steadily increase in number and whose outpatient department steadily loses money. In big cities, however, there often is no family doctor for this group. A great many children of such families can be handled in Well Baby Clinics. In the state of Maryland, this is usually the best disposition for them: the city Well Baby Clinics, on the other hand, are staffed largely by a rotating group of physicians, and although they are highly efficient, it is not possible for them to maintain the warm relationship a family doctor can provide. (See Table VI-3.)

Group D has had a bad hospital experience. The child from this group has a severe chronic disease such as nephritis and has a prolonged illness ahead. His home is good.

The parents need, and should be given, detailed instructions. At the same time they should be allowed a great deal of guided freedom for imaginative development of their own. Home visiting both by the family doctor and by the public health nurse is extremely useful in this group, and should, if possible, be organized on a co-operative basis before the child is discharged. The arrange-

TABLE VI-3

GROUP C: BENIGN HOSPITALIZATION, POOR HOME

I. Emotionally poor home
  A. Utilize family doctor
  B. Be available, noncritical
  C. Relinquish hold

II. Economically poor home
  A. Utilize all available social agencies
  B. Relinquish hold

III. Emotionally and economically poor home
  A. Work with responsible figure and mother
  B. Follow-up by family doctor

ment of home schooling before the child leaves is exceedingly important.

I am delighted to hear about telephone hookups from the classroom into the home. I would also suggest that teachers encourage their pupils to visit home-bound children and to think of ways to help them.

It has been pointed out that since discussion of sex is no longer taboo (and, indeed, is virtually unavoidable at all times and in all places), it has been replaced as a taboo subject by death. The lack of sympathy and understanding and the lack of recognition of the necessity of mourning are examples of this new taboo. Another subject that is not realistically discussed in our society is chronic sickness. A patient who is chronically ill is popularly assumed by most people to be some kind of malingerer! The assumption is very generally made that if he would only pull himself together he would soon be out working again. When the patient is a child, it is often assumed that the parents are malingerers or overprotective.

These situations do exist, but we cannot be blind to the fact the chronically ill need visiting and work and should not be treated as outcasts.

For Group D children, parents' groups may be helpful; so may leukemia groups, muscular dystrophy groups, and so forth. Such groups are undoubtedly helpful in the field of mental retardation.

Hospital visits for Group D will be frequent; they should be brief, pleasant, and cheerful for all concerned. The child and his family should receive continued support from these visits by a small, well-organized medical group. Physicians play key roles in this group. Although two or three will probably treat and come to know the particular patient and his parents, one physician should have the major responsibility for each individual patient. The value of follow-up visits can be greatly increased by nonmedical personnel: the public health nurse, the physiotherapist, the social worker, the nurse, and the receptionist. The concept of this medical group as a united one is not original, but it is very difficult to insure in a teaching institution. Nonetheless, a constant, conscious effort must be made by all concerned. This group should be receptive to fresh ideas. At the same time it should not vacillate between one method of treatment and another, between one psychological approach and another. An atmosphere of cheerful calm as well as professional unity should prevail and be conveyed to the parents. (See Table VI-4.)

TABLE VI-4

GROUP D: BAD HOSPITAL EXPERIENCE, GOOD HOME,
PROLONGED ILLNESS AHEAD

I.   Detailed instructions, with personal elasticity

II.   Home visits, home teacher

III.   Support
    A.   Frequent, brief, pleasant visits
    B.   Clubs
    C.   Continued support by small united group

IV.   Coherent plan with calm affect

I do not think the handling of this particular group differs according to the clinical prognosis for the child. The situation is much more painful and difficult when death appears inevitable, as in leukemia or muscular dystrophy. The basic approach to the child and the parents is different only in the quantity, not in the quality, of support required.

Group E is that in which both home and hospital experience are bad. At home the child is grossly neglected or badly treated; the parents are psychotic, alcoholic, or gravely disturbed. The situation unfortunately is by no means as rare as it is generally thought to be. To my knowledge we have two such patients in the hospital, both victims of very gross and terrible neglect, with all the appalling psychological damage this treatment causes. These children are completely withdrawn. They are devoid of what psychologists call "stimulation" but what can also be referred to, perhaps more truly, as a lack of love, or, occasionally, as positive cruelty.

We have not yet learned to handle this group well. It should be investigated while the child is hospitalized. Ideally a major conference should be held on each child. This conference should include the people involved in the child's hospital care, the social worker who has investigated the case, and the social agency to whom this problem family will be referred.

Whenever there appears to be any reasonable hope of doing so, every effort should be made to improve the home situation. Although there are many cases in which this is impossible, we have not really explored the possibility of re-educating and re-orienting some of these delinquent parents. In order to do this, we need a different approach. We need people who will visit in the home and actively help the mother in the daily routines.

I feel great sympathy for an unmarried Negro girl of twenty who has four children by different men. When she talks to the average social worker or the usual white intern or resident doctor, she knows very little of their world. If she is intelligent, as many are, she recognizes quite clearly that they know nothing of hers. This is the appalling emotional and cultural poverty that we in the hospitals must help dissipate.

Although we must not assume that every child who comes into the hospital will go back to a clean, pleasant, affectionate home, neither must we be so blind as to believe that affection and good care is necessarily lacking in a family constellation that is unfamiliar. It is always pleasanter and easier to work with cheerful, co-operative parents whose children have been cured than it is to deal with poorly motivated parents whose child is still sick, may continue through childhood to be an invalid, and, one has reason to fear, may grow up to be as poor a parent as his own. (See Table VI-5.)

TABLE VI-5
GROUP E: BAD HOSPITAL EXPERIENCE, BAD HOME

I.   Investigate realistically while child is in hospital

II. Improve home situation if possible

III. New approaches need developing

In summary then, outpatient follow-up of children is extraordinarily important. There is a time to hold on to patients, and often we do not keep them long enough; and there is a time to release patients, and sometimes we do not free them rapidly enough. I have discussed these subjects rather than the question of how to tell the mother exactly how much digitalis to give the child or how to explain to her what digitalis is. These are very important points and should be handled by the nurse or physician. The other aspects of posthospital care are the responsibility of the hospital staff as a whole and are not yet adequately evaluated or adequately handled. In some respects this reflects the inadequacy of our hospital administration setup and the tunnel vision that hospital life induces. But there are more fundamental reasons. Our inadequacy is a reflection of a general social failure to accept and recognize personal responsibility for the presence of suffering and death, even in an institution as brightly colored and as academically adorned as the Children's Medical and Surgical Center.

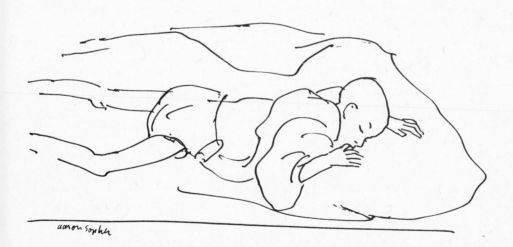

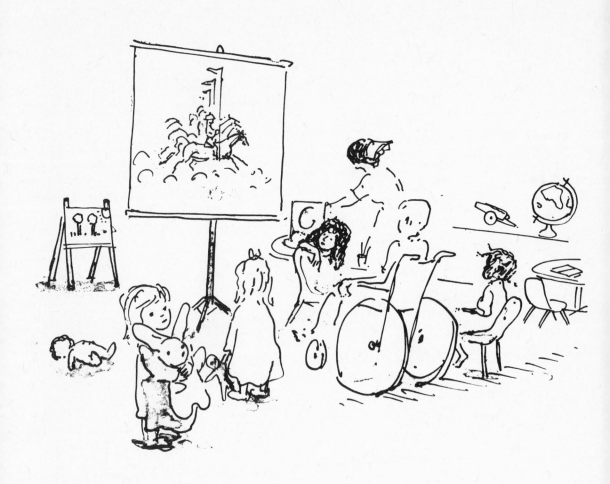

Chapter VII

THE HELEN SCHNETZER CHILD LIFE PROGRAM

Robert H. Dombro, M.A., and Barbara Schuyler Haas, B.S.*

The depth of interest and consideration for the ill and hospitalized child and his family is a comparatively new development in the field of pediatrics. Although many thoughtful physicians have noted with grave concern the adverse effects of illness and hospitalization on their young patients, little was done to change the management of pediatric cases until studies by Prugh and others appeared in the pediatric and psychiatric journals in the early 1930s. Since that time, hospitals across the country have slowly altered their traditional handling of a child's hospitalization and are adopting more constructive measures for the emotional and physical well-being of the child and his family.

An important step in implementing the theories of good hospital management of children is to have a permanent staff actively engaged in the day-to-day programing for patients. They will have concern both for the growth and developmental needs of the child and for the emotional aspects of the experiences that confront the child and his family. A few hospitals now have such specialized personnel who direct programs varying in range and depth of development. Included among them is the Child Life Program in the Children's Medical and Surgical Center of The Johns Hopkins Hospital.

During the summer of 1944, Miss Onica Prall, Head of the Child Develop-

* Director, The Child Life Program, The Johns Hopkins Hospital.

ment Department of Hood College, directed several of her senior students in a volunteer demonstration program for patients in the ward area of the Harriet Lane Home. Their approach to the child was through play, and the value of providing play activities was quickly appreciated by the nursing and medical staffs. Upon the recommendation of Miss Helen Schnetzer, then supervisor of pediatric nursing, and with the full approval of the professor of pediatrics and the hospital administrator, the program became a permanent one and was known as "Play Activities." A staff of preschool teachers was engaged, and the program was extended to include private patients in the Harriet Lane Home and the pediatric-surgical patients in the Halsted Pavillion. The Women's Board of the Hospital provided important financial support for this new undertaking.

As the needs of the hospitalized child became better understood, work with children was broadened to include a school program. Recognition of the importance of parents in child care brought about a concerted effort to include them in activities. This expanded endeavor was renamed "The Child Life Program" by Dr. Robert E. Cooke, as defining more closely the concept of family-centered pediatric care that the Children's Center now provides. Simultaneously, the scope of the program and its role in the hospital have also widened with the realization that a meaningful contribution may be made by its staff to the education of medical and nursing students, technicians, and others in training for work with children.

The Child Life Program today is an integral part of the medical, surgical, and nursing services in the Children's Center. Administratively it is within the Division of Nursing in the Department of Pediatrics. The permanent staff includes a director, a supervisor, and preschool, elementary, and secondary school teachers, all with either bachelor's or master's degrees in child development or education. A strong background in the field of human development is important, and a deep concern for people is essential. Staff members recognize the potential adverse effects of illness and hospitalization on the behavior of both children and their families but also believe that a hospital experience can be a strengthening one for the whole family. Their work with children shows an appreciation of the need to provide a setting that encourages the continuation of normal growth and development. The staff provides important continuity in the hospital life of a child who otherwise meets an endless stream of new personnel in the course of each day. An orientation to the hospital and the program is given new staff members, and continued inservice education is accomplished through staff meetings in which patients and planning are discussed and journal articles are reviewed.

The Women's Board continues to be the major financial support of the program; in addition, several nursing service and education positions have been transferred to the Child Life Program and have enabled its staff to grow. Salaries are in line with the local salary scale for teachers in the public schools. The program is conducted seven days a week, twelve months of the year.

The vast majority of hospitalized children and adolescents, age two to eighteen, are included in the program. Most activities are centered in the play-school-dining areas on the fourth, seventh, eighth, and ninth floors of the Children's Medical and Surgical Center. These areas are designed to accommodate beds and wheelchairs and have a center folding wall that enables the staff to divide the rooms and conduct separate programs for preschool and school-age children. The areas are located next to the pantries so that lunch and dinner can be easily served to groups of children.

Equipment and creative materials are chosen to stimulate normal development at the various age levels as well as to encourage the expression of emotions. A housekeeping corner, furniture and toys, solid blocks, puzzles, manipulative toys, puppets, board games, water trays, easels and poster paints, fingerpaints, clay, crayons, and collage and craft materials are provided. Animal cages and aquariums house the hospital pets; bulletin boards display children's works of art. Telephones are available for calls home. Large windows provide a spectacular view of the city skyline and changes in weather. Schoolroom sections are equipped with the familiar blackboards, flags, and globes. An outdoor play deck, accessible from the chronic care center on the fourth floor, has swings, a sandbox, a fish pond, and planting space. A grassy area in the center of the Hospital complex with sliding boards, swings, and a picnic area is available to the children, as well as a gymnasium in case of bad weather. Outdoor equipment includes bicycles and tricycles, wagons, a badminton set, horseshoes, balls and bats, pails, and other suitable toys.

A major concern of the Child Life Program Staff is the creation of a setting in which children feel free to explore, to investigate, to experiment, to choose activities, and to express themselves. Although the atmosphere is a permissive one, limits are necessary for security and welfare of the children. The recognition of individual problems by the staff, demonstrated through use of materials, may lead to referrals to other hospital services or play an important part in future guidance plans. The program for the preschool child is essentially the same as one in a typical nursery school, with modifications for the broad age span and the constantly changing group.

It is unrealistic to think that the developmental need for intellectual stimulation can be met without providing a school program. Therefore teachers are hired by the hospital so that both acutely and chronically ill children, regardless of the length of stay, are eligible for participation. Each child is accepted on his present level of ability; the result is a "one-room schoolhouse" with its wide range of ages and grades. Special materials such as programed reading are used. Small classes make it possible to give individual help to children with academic deficiencies. The fostering of a positive attitude toward education is another goal. With their doctors' permission, children attend class in the schoolroom in the morning. Patients confined to their rooms are visited by a staff member in the morning and tutored in the afternoon. Arts and crafts activities are correlated with social studies instruction and holiday activities.

A children's library was established several years ago, and children of all ages make weekly library visits. The older children use its reference books in their schoolwork; leisure-time books and picture books can be borrowed. Teachers of all groups find materials to supplement their teaching. The Enoch Pratt Library is a source of additional books as well as films, which are shown once a week. Holidays bring parties, and community groups frequently provide special treats: magicians, puppet shows, clowns, and concerts. Summer cookouts and picnics are popular. Children and their families often attend Sunday morning church services held by the hospital chaplain.

Programing on the long-term fourth floor differs from that on the other acute floors. Patients here are hospitalized for many months, and more effort is made to vary their experiences. They wear street clothes, and excursions to different parts of the hospital and to neighborhood stores are frequent. The educational program keeps the children at their grade level and often utilizes textbooks from their home schools. Special considerations have been made for the adolescent patients on the ninth floor: lounge-type furniture and equipment as well as a set of ground rules reflect the needs of this important age group. Schoolwork usually consists of the patient's assignments from his own school. Weekly sessions with a social group worker gives the adolescent an opportunity to talk freely about his illness and his hospitalization.

As increasing numbers of patients are being seen on an outpatient basis in our "inner" cities; outpatient departments are assuming more responsibility in the total care of patients and their families. Hospitals have been pinpointed as key agencies in the fight against debilitating social problems as well as disease. Sensitive staff, working with children and their families in a nonmedical capacity, are often able to identify developmental lags, emotional difficulties, or financial needs and can contribute to the total planning of the family unit. Emphasis is placed on gaining rapport with the family to develop the concept of the hospital as a warm, accepting place where staff is interested in the well-being of the child and his family. There are two outpatient areas staffed by members of the Child Life Program. The equipment and activities are similar to those on the inpatient floors: toys and games and creative educational and recreational materials for many different age groups. Family members accompanying the patient are encouraged to participate while the child is waiting to be treated by the medical staff. Child Life Program Staff members also provide service to several of the pediatric specialty clinics.

Older children are occasionally admitted to nonpediatric areas of the hospital and are referred to the Child Life Program by their doctors or nurses. A staff member visits and supplies books and other materials, and whenever possible, these children are taken to play-school-dining areas for activities. Children hospitalized for more than eight weeks are eligible for a schoolteacher from the Baltimore Department of Education.

Parents are very much in evidence in all parts of the Children's Center, and the value of their presence is recognized by the staff. Many mothers live in the hospital during their child's hospitalization. Child Life Program staff members work closely with the nurse who co-ordinates the living-in program for mothers (or fathers), and an exchange of observations and information is invaluable. Families are encouraged to participate in activities in the play-school-dining areas, where they often find an oasis of "normal" activity in an otherwise foreign land. Like their children, they may be able to express their feelings more easily in a nonthreatening setting. Parents of chronically ill and handicapped children have an opportunity to see their children in better perspective, under the supervision of an accepting and understanding staff. They have the opportunity to see good guidance techniques and to become acquainted with equipment and creative materials suitable for various age levels. Observation of the school program relieves much of the concern the overanxious parent may have regarding time missed from the home school. In the overprotective parent it may also foster a healthier attitude toward the importance of school attendance. The Child Life Program has prepared a booklet "You And Your Child At The Children's Center" to familiarize parents and their children with the regulations and procedures encountered during hospitalization.

The Child Life Program is keenly aware of the possibilities in a teaching hospital of affecting the thinking of the many staffs who come in contact with the child. Discussions are held, in co-operation with department heads, with house staff in pediatrics and pediatric surgery. There are meetings with the fourth-year medical students during their five-week experience in pediatrics. The effects of hospitalization on children and their families, as well as the organization and role of the Child Life Program, are discussed.

The educational program for nursing students is a more extensive one. A pre-clinical course in human development is taught by the supervisor of the program, and an additional five hours in child growth and development and children's play, emphasizing the effects of illness and hospitalization on normal growth and development, are given during the thirteen-week pediatric clinical experience. Nursing students spend two weeks of their time in pediatrics in the Child Life Program. After an introduction to their assigned area, a session on the school program, a class on crafts and creative materials, and a discussion on the basic principles of guiding children, they observe the teachers and participate in an assistant's capacity. Students have an opportunity to work with younger and older children, in groups in the playrooms and schoolrooms, as well as individually with children confined to their rooms. Their observations are discussed daily with the teachers. During the second week of participation, students present an oral behavioral study on one of the children with whom they have worked, discussing the child from the medical, social, emotional, and educational viewpoints, comparing him with the textbook picture of a child his age, and suggesting a plan for his guidance. Notes of these studies are filed on cards for future student reference as well as for information on the child in the case of readmission. Students, under supervision, staff the play-school-dining areas on weekends. Students wear a Child Life Program badge to identify them as a part of the program. A member of the program staff co-ordinates the student's experience and, with the co-operation of the teachers, evaluates her performance. Her grade earned is part of her final grade in pediatric practice. Other services include a three-month training period for college graduates and upper classmen with appropriate academic backgrounds, a thirty-hour fieldwork experience for a group of Goucher College education majors, and many discussion-observations for undergraduate and graduate students from other schools of nursing.

Many children are in great need of individual attention: someone to play a game, to feed them, to read a story, or just an unhurried someone to listen. A welcome addition to the regular staff are the volunteers, who give hundreds of hours each year. After an initial screening by the Hospital Director of Volunteers and an orientation to the general hospital policies and procedures, the volunteer who has shown an interest in work with children is given an additional orientation to the Child Life Program. This includes an explanation of a volunteer's duties, isolation techniques, principles in guiding children, and a brief demonstration of basic craft materials. Volunteers sign in at the Child Life Program Office and are assigned to an area where they are needed. Staff members then guide them in their work with individual children confined to their rooms or with groups in the play-school-dining areas. More experienced volunteers are often sent to work with toddlers on the fifth floor or the sixth floor Intensive Care Unit. A group of volunteers under the guidance of a former children's librarian established and maintain the children's library and book cart service for children unable to leave their floors. Another group has regular puppet-making sessions with children on the long-term floor, while another gives weekly puppet shows in both inpatient and outpatient areas. Evening volunteers are supervised by an afternoon-evening staff member. An extensive program with junior volunteers is conducted during the summer months. After a Red Cross First Aid Course and an orientation to the Child Life Program, juniors participate in the program and hold weekly discussions on the effects of illness and hospitalization on children and related subjects. They are responsible for an oral review of an article on the hospitalization of children as well as a written report on some phase of their own experience. All volunteers working in the Child Life Program wear Child Life Program badges in addition to regular hospital volunteer badges.

Good communication among all staffs is a necessity if the hospital expects to meet the over-all needs of the child and his family. It is often difficult to accomplish this on a busy floor with the constantly changing shifts of nurses and aides, the added complication of rotating house staff, and the large number of private pediatricians. The morning report that is given to the Child Life Program staff by the head nurses is invaluable. Such information as the physical condition of each child, his diet, scheduled treatment or surgical procedures, which children are to be discharged, how many admissions are expected, and any other pertinent information concerning the floor are needed to plan the activities of the day. This is a time when staff can share observations of children with the nurses and have their questions answered. Histories are available to the staff, and contributions to the daily report sheets are made. The staff attend floor team conferences and take part in the weekly multidisciplinary conferences on the fourth and ninth floors. They comment on the chronically ill child or adolescent from their special viewpoint and present problems parents may have revealed. Communication on an administrative level is of equal importance to the effectiveness and growth of the program. Representation in the Children's Medical and Surgical Center Care Committee, attendance at head nurses' and supervisors' meetings, and participation in the pediatric educational group staff meetings are valuable in maintaining a close working relationship with all personnel concerned with the child and his family. Frequent professional contacts with social service, child psychiatry, and occupational therapy are important.

The Child Life Program has sponsored several lecture series in an effort to kindle community interest in the adverse effect of hospitalization on the child's psyche and to emphasize the importance of instituting programs like that at the Hopkins for counteracting this aspect of illness. A 16mm film entitled *A Family Goes to the Hospital* has been produced from a thirty-minute television Johns Hopkins Review Program and is available from the Maryland State Department of Health. Staff members frequently speak to church, education, and child study groups. Nationally, the program was host to a three-day conference for people conducting comparable programs in hospitals in the United States and Canada.

Future plans include an extension of the program and full-time staff to the floor for infants and toddlers and the Intensive Care Unit. A permanent home for the library and a librarian are needed. A supply of trained people is imperative to meet the increasing demands of hospitals wanting to establish programs, and an extensive training program to accommodate many students must be developed. A booklet designed especially for children, to supplement the information now given parents, is important; so is a film to be used in community and training sessions.

Unfortunately, the results of a recent survey of children's hospitals and pediatric sections of general hospitals in the United States and Canada indicate that there are still too many facilities for children which underestimate the importance of providing a similar or modified program (see Appendixes A and B). There are still too many hospitals that do not believe that the hospitalization of a child merits the effort necessary to provide total care. There are still too many hospitals that shun the family. Such conditions should not be tolerated, and they will not be if pediatricians and pediatric surgeons speak out and voice their displeasure.

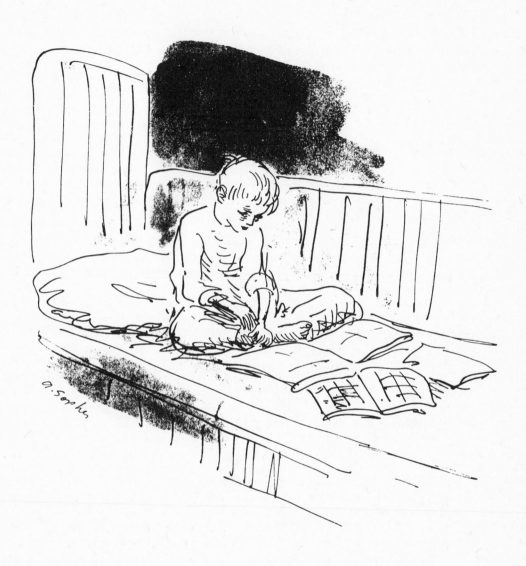

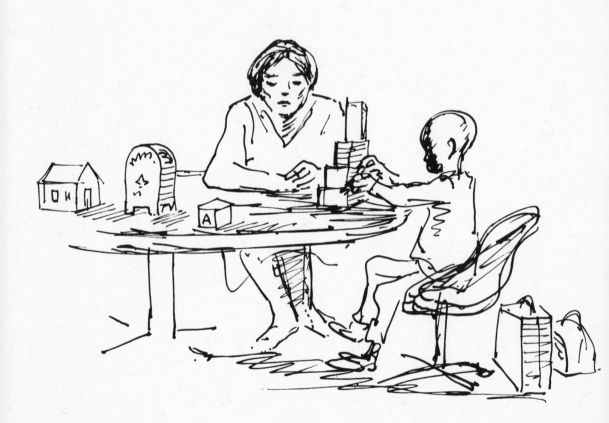

CHILD LIFE PROGRAMS IN NINETY-ONE CHILDREN'S HOSPITALS IN THE UNITED STATES AND CANADA

Robert H. Dombro, M.A.

INTRODUCTION

Pediatricians, pediatric surgeons, and other hospital staffs who wish to improve the care of hospitalized children and their families may be interested in the data collected by means of a questionnaire sent by the Children's Medical and Surgical Center to 132 children's hospitals in the United States and Canada to ascertain the development of Child Life Programs. All hospitals categorized as facilities for children in the *Journal of the American Hospital Association,* August, 1964, Part Two, were included—with the exception of psychiatric hospitals. Of these, 91—69 per cent—returned their questionnaires, completed to varying degrees; 41 did not reply. Hospitals were classified for this survey according to the length of stay of the patient population: long-term hospitals accommodate children for an average hospitalization of more than two weeks, short-term hospitals, for two weeks or less. Because of the lack of completed questionnaires uniform totals were not possible for all aspects of Child Life programing. Sufficient information was available, however, to give the reader an idea of the practices of children's hospitals in the area of Child Life Programs.

Questionnaires were addressed to the administrators of hospitals, since it was not known which hospitals had staff working specifically with children in a Child

Life Program capacity. While more than 50 per cent of the returns were signed by administrators and only 14 per cent by directors of Child Life Programs, there was evidence that most of the responses were the combined efforts of several hospital staffs.

Programs are loosely defined as staff actively engaged in meeting growth and developmental needs of children. Of the 91 hospitals 69—76 per cent—stated that they have programs; in 22, children are cared for by nursing staff but there is no program.

Pediatricians, psychiatrists, surgeons, social workers, nurses, and educators have reported on the potential psychological dangers of hospital experiences and have repeatedly stressed the values of providing opportunities for continual growth and development in the hospital environment, regardless of the length of stay or the severity of the medical problem. Yet more than half of the 22 children's hospitals without programs replied that they felt no need for them, often justifying this with the fact that the average length of stay is under a week. It is gratifying to note that 8 of these 22 hospitals do recognize the need for a program and desire to establish one.

Judging by the vast array of names of programs and by the variety of hospital departments under which programs were placed administratively, there is no uniform concept of the unique role of Child Life Programs among hospitals. There is no single established profession engaged in directing such hospital programs. Hospitals whose programs are directly responsible to the department of pediatrics or to the administration see them most clearly as separate groups contributing to the care of the child and his family and not as adjuncts to existing professions.

Of the 9,189 children in 88 hospitals, including both long- and short-term facilities, less than one-fourth (not all hospitals answered this question) are provided with any sort of an educational experience. Most long- and short-term hospitals have acceptable child-teacher ratios. One wonders, however, what sort of academic accomplishment is possible in the long-term hospital that reports 1 teacher for every 25 to 30 children.

It was difficult to judge the quality of their books and the actual use of them by the children from the figures on libraries. Although 52 hospitals reported libraries, only 13 have money budgeted for the purchase of books and only 16 have full- or part-time librarians. There is a total of 46,500 volumes in 31 hospitals. There does not appear to be sufficient staff to provide an adequate library setting for the majority of hospitalized children.

Although more than half the responding hospitals reported recreational staff, in most of the long-term hospitals there was only 1 staff member per 40 to 100 children. There is 1 short-term hospital with 1 staff person for 250 children. Surely a facility of this size should be aware of the effects of hospitalization and the value of providing recreation programs. Such inability to supply adequate staffing is inexcusable and should not be tolerated by the community at large. Only a few hospitals seem to have sufficient staff to meet children's recreational needs.

Twenty-four of the hospitals have Child Life staff with bachelor's and master's degrees; the average salary is $5,338 a year. This is extremely low and indicates perhaps that such personnel is considered "extra" by some hospital administrators rather than essential for total child care.

The survey does not show how many schools of nursing were affiliated with the various hospitals, but 31 of the hospital Child Life Programs are used to educate nursing student groups, and their training includes supervised participation.

Hospitals have long been aware of the benefits of an extensive volunteer program. The large number of paid directors of volunteers probably attests to hospital and community interest in giving time to the care of children. The list of volunteer tasks is an excellent guide for the imaginative use of volunteers in hospital settings.

Both long- and short-term hospitals provide space for children's activities, although almost one-third of the facilities are used for other purposes. Of the responding hospitals, almost 40 per cent reported that these areas are used without supervision. Most of these hospitals provide full-day programs, 5 days a week.

Twenty-one hospitals reported facilities for mothers to live in, but the small number of mothers who actually take advantage of this service indicates both that its real value to children and mothers is not understood and that medical and nursing staffs do not encourage use of the facilities. Possibly many mothers are even unaware of them and thus of the benefits they and their children may derive.

Continuing contact with home during a long hospitalization is important; yet more than half the responding long-term hospitals restrict visiting hours to less than 4 hours a day, some to 1 hour a week. Two short-term hospitals restrict visiting, but a large number of these hospitals show more concern than long-term hospitals for the presence of parents as well as flexibility in their management of patients.

Almost three times as many hospital staffs rated their understanding and acceptance of Child Life Programs as "excellent" and "very good," as compared to staffs rating programs "good" or "poor." This is an indication that where programs exist they have the support of other disciplines for their individual contributions to the well-being of the child and his family. Surgeons, particularly orthopedic surgeons, were the least accepting.

This report is concerned with a survey of Child Life Programs[1] in children's hospitals in the United States and Canada. A 17-page questionnaire was sent to the administrators of 132 of these hospitals; 91—69 per cent—replied. General children's hospitals, orthopedic children's hospitals, and chronic disease and/or convalescent hospitals were included in the survey; children's psychiatric hospitals were not.[2]

The survey attempted to gain information about 14 areas:

1. Number of Child Life Programs
2. Names of Child Life Programs
3. Placement of Child Life Programs in hospital structure
4. Children and staff in educational programs
5. Hours of school per day
6. Children's libraries
7. Children and staff in recreational programs
8. Salaries of staff
9. Student nurse involvement
10. Volunteer participation
11. Space allotted for Child Life Programs
12. Mothers' living-in programs
13. Visiting hours
14. Rating of Child Life Programs by other hospital staffs

The questionnaire was answered as follows:

Answered by		Per cent
administrators	52	57
directors of Child Life Programs	13	14
medical directors	7	8
nursing director	1	1
no signatures	18	20

[1] The program at the Children's Medical and Surgical Center, The Johns Hopkins Hospital, is called the Child Life Program. Other hospitals use other names for such programs; these are listed in the section "Names of Child Life Programs."

[2] A total of 9,189 children were in 88 of 91 hospitals when the survey was taken; 3 hospitals did not report their census. Fifty-three hospitals reported 1,697 beds for prematures, infants, and toddlers; 38 hospitals did not report number of beds for these patients. The survey was taken in February, 1966; the report completed in July, 1966. The questionnaire used for the survey was compiled by Mrs. Barbara S. Haas, Supervisor, Child Life Program, The Johns Hopkins Hospital.

Hospitals were classified as long-term or short-term; long-term hospitals accommodate children two weeks or more; short-term hospitals, two weeks or less. Of the 91, 49—54 per cent—are long-term; 42—46 per cent—are short-term.

1. NUMBER OF CHILD LIFE PROGRAMS

Of the 91 hospitals that answered, 69—76 per cent—have Child Life Programs; 22—24 per cent—have no program. The latter group explained the absence of a program as follows:[3]

    13 do not feel the need.
     8 do not have sufficient funds.
     5 do not have knowledge in the field.
     3 give other reasons.

Asked if they desired to establish programs, they replied as follows:

     8 desire to establish programs.
    13 do not desire to establish programs.
     1 desires to establish a program possibly.

2. NAMES OF CHILD LIFE PROGRAMS

The names used to describe Child Life Programs are numerous. Of the 91 hospitals 48 reporting programs have a name; 3 do not; 18 did not answer the question. The 48 programs are designated as follows:[4]

School	12
Occupational therapy	9
Recreational therapy	8
Recreation	2
Different names	17

---

[3] Some hospitals gave more than one reason.

[4] The different names included: Children's Activity Department; Children's Activity Service; Child Care; Child Development Unit–School; Extra Curricular Activities; Formal Education–Preschool; Group Activities Department; Group Work Program–Intramural School; Institutional School–House Parent Recreation; Play Program–School; Recreational Activities; Recreation Department–Play Lady Program; Recreation Program–Play School; Rehabilitation–Recreation Program; Residential Treatment Department; Special Education Program; Special Education–Recreation Program.

3. PLACEMENT OF CHILD LIFE PROGRAMS IN HOSPITAL STRUCTURE

Supervision of Child Life Programs varies. The majority is either autonomous or supervised by or incorporated in the occupational therapy departments of the hospital:[5]

Supervision	No. of programs
autonomous	12
occupational therapy	12
nursing service	7
administration	6
child psychiatry	4
department of pediatrics	2
physical therapy	2
social service	2
county, city, or state departments of education	33

4. CHILDREN AND STAFF IN EDUCATIONAL PROGRAMS

Of the 9,189 children reported in the 88 hospitals, an educational program is provided for 2,090. Of the 49 long-term hospitals, 36 reported specific details about their education programs; 17 of 42 short-term hospitals reported details:

	No. of children	Education staff	No. of children per teacher (average)
Long-term hospitals 36	1765	208	8
Short-term hospitals 17	325	30	11

In long-term hospitals number of staff members per child ranges from 1 member for 1 to 5 children to 1 member for 25 to 30 children.

No. of long-term hospitals	No. of children per teacher
5	1–5
15	6–10
11	11–15
4	16–20
1	25–30

[5] Several of the programs reported that the teaching personnel was usually, though not always, responsible to the local department of education; consequently, some personnel had dual supervision.

94

In short-term hospitals the range is from 1 member for 1 to 5 children to 1 member for 45 to 50 children.

No. of short-term hospitals	No. of children per teacher
3	1–5
6	6–10
5	11–15
1	16–20
1	25–30
1	45–50

5. HOURS OF SCHOOL PER DAY

Of the 91 hospitals, 58 replied to this question. Of these, 53 have formal education programs and 5[6] have informal programs. The daily average is 5.1 hours.

No. of hospitals	Hours of school per day	Per cent
7	2.5–3	12
6	3–4	10
17	4–5	29
22	5–6	38
5	6–7	9
1	7–7.5	2

6. CHILDREN'S LIBRARIES

There is a total of 52 children's libraries in the 91 hospitals—30 in the 49 long-term hospitals, 22 in the 42 short-term hospitals—and a total of 46,500 volumes (only 31 hospitals reported number of volumes). Of the long-term hospitals, 8 have a library budget, 17 have none, and 5 did not answer the question. Of the short-term hospitals, 5 have a budget, 14 have none, and 3 did not answer the question. Of the long-term hospitals, 10 have librarians (9 part-time, 1 full-time), 17 have none, and 3 did not answer the question. Of the short-term hospitals, 6 have librarians (5 part-time, 1 full-time), 13 have none, and 3 did not answer the question.

	No. of libraries	No. of volumes
Long-term hospitals		
49	30	26,850
Short-term hospitals		
42	22	19,650

---

[6] These were not conducted by teachers.

7. CHILDREN AND STAFF IN RECREATIONAL PROGRAMS

Of the 9,189 children reported in 88 hospitals, recreation programs are provided for 5,690. Of these hospitals, 45 reported as follows:

	No. of children	No. of staff	No. of children per member
Long-term hospitals 26	1,982	90	22
Short-term hospitals 19	3,708	75	49

In long-term hospitals number of staff members per child ranges from 1 member for 1 to 10 children to 1 member for 91 to 100 children.

No. of long-term hospitals	No. of children per staff member
3	1–10
4	11–20
3	21–30
2	31–40
1	41–50
6	51–60
3	61–70
2	71–80
1	81–90
1	91–100

In short-term hospitals the range is from 1 recreation staff member for 20 to 30 children to 1 member for 251 to 260 children.

No. of short-term hospitals	No. of children per staff member
4	20–30
6	31–40
3	41–50
3	71–80
1	91–100
1	171–180
1	251–260

8. SALARIES OF STAFF

Salaries for full-time personnel conducting Child Life Programs range from $2,300 to $10,500 annually. Personnel range from recent high school graduates to those with master's degrees in education, child development, and recreation. There are personnel with master's degrees in 3 hospitals and with bachelor's degrees in 21 hospitals. Those conducting the recreation programs are usually paid by the hospital; those conducting the education programs are usually paid by the local department of education, and their salaries are determined by the salary scale of the local department.

The following salary information is for personnel conducting recreation programs who may also have responsibility for co-ordinating the education program within the hospital. Of the 91 hospitals, 29 provided salary figures: 18 gave a scale and 11 gave only one figure.

Scale	*One figure*
$2,300–$6,000	$2,400
2,400– 4,800	4,068
2,616– 6,300	4,200
2,700– 4,800	4,500
3,000– 5,000	5,000
3,234– 4,773	5,000
3,900– 6,760	5,280
3,900– 7,280	5,280
4,000– 7,200	5,400
4,100– 6,900	7,200
4,200– 8,300	10,000
4,500– 7,150	
4,804– 7,050	
5,000– 7,000	
5,000– 7,500	
5,100– 7,500	
5,400– 8,500	
6,000–10,500	

The average annual salary for the 18 hospitals is $5,374; the average for the 11 is $5,302.

9. STUDENT NURSE INVOLVEMENT

Of the 49 long-term hospitals, 15 report that student nurses are involved in Child Life Programs; 16 of the 42 short-term hospitals report student nurses involved. The length of time spent in the programs varies from 2 hours to 2 weeks. Of the 31 hospitals reporting student nurse involvement, student nurses observe the program in 7; observe and participate in 12; participate in 9; 3 hospitals did not answer the question. In 17 of the programs, student nurses are supervised by nursing personnel; in 9 programs supervision is provided by educational and recreational personnel; 3 hospitals report that student nurses are supervised by nursing and education-recreational personnel. In 2 hospitals student nurses provided educational and recreational service as part of total nursing care.

Special classes for student nurses include growth and development, philosophy of recreation, behavior of the hospitalized child, orientation to play programs, rehabilitation of handicapped children, and play for the ill child. Assignments include conducting a play project, giving case presentations, writing a developmental paper, and choosing toys for patients of different ages.

10. VOLUNTEER PARTICIPATION

Of the 49 long-term hospitals, 14 have paid directors of volunteers; of the 42 short-term hospitals, 19 have paid directors. These 33 hospitals reported 1,592 adult volunteers annually: 1,488 women—93 per cent—and 104 men—7 per cent. A total of 867 junior volunteers (Candy Stripers)—756 girls, or 87 per cent, and 111 boys, or 13 per cent—work in 30 of the 33 hospitals. The majority of junior volunteers worked only in the summer. In-service training programs vary from 1 to 30 hours, with several hospitals reporting continuous on-the-job training.

There were 60 volunteer tasks mentioned:

arranging parties	ceramics	escorting to school
baking	child care	feeding
bathing	club work	games
bedside recreation	crafts	group activities
bird identification	dancing	hand activity development
car rides	entertaining	handiwork

holding	O.T. aide	spelling
homework	outdoor field trips	supervising games
horticulture	piano	swimming
knitting	play	taking children for walks
leatherwork	playroom activity	teaching
letter writing	play school	toileting
library assistant	preschool activities	transporting to x-ray therapy
library cart	P.T. aide	tricycle riding
listening to reading	reading	tutoring
loaning toy carts	refreshments	typing
mail distribution	rocking	walking training
model building	scout assistance	ward clerking
music appreciation	selecting TV-radio program	wheelchair rides
music therapy	showing films	woodwork

11. SPACE ALLOTTED FOR CHILD LIFE PROGRAMS

A total of 53 hospitals reported 138 areas designated for programs: 32 of the 49 long-term hospitals and 21 of the 42 short-term hospitals. Of these 112 are playrooms. Other areas are schoolrooms, gymnasiums, swimming pools, libraries, hobby rooms, and outdoor playgrounds. The areas are open from 2 to 14 hours a day, an average of 6.3 hours a day, Monday through Friday, with 3 hospitals reporting a 6-day program, including Saturdays and 1 a 7-day program.

Of the 138 areas, 101 have specific program hours; of these, 58 are available for programming 6 hours or more; 43 were available 6 hours or less. Areas are never used without supervision in 31 hospitals and are used without supervision in 18. Of the 138, 79 are not shared with other programs, 45 are; for 14 areas there was no information regarding sharing.

Square footage of 108 areas ranges from 100 square feet to 10,000 square feet and totals 123,625 square feet, an average of 1,145 square feet per area. Of the 108 areas, 24 have more than 1,145 square feet; 84 have less.

12. MOTHERS' LIVING-IN PROGRAMS

There are facilities for mothers' living in with their hospitalized children in 21 hospitals: 1 in the 49 long-term hospitals and 20 in the 42 short-term hospitals. The number of mothers living in ranges from 1 to 12 daily. Costs range from no charge to $5.00 per day. In one hospital, mothers who take part in the Family Participation Unit, where they provide nursing care, reduce their children's hospital rate by $3.00 per day.

Of the 21, 11 provide living-in facilities for mothers of all economic levels; 7 have facilities only for mothers of private patients; 3 did not answer the question. Whether or not mothers live in is determined by physicians at 7 hospitals, by physicians and nurses at 2, by mothers at 3 hospitals, by the business department at 1, and by the program director at 1; 7 hospitals did not answer the question.

13. VISITING HOURS

There were 55 replies to the question on visiting hours: 32 from long-term hospitals, 23 from short-term. Visiting hours range from liberal—4 hours or more per day—to restrictive—less than 4 hours per day. The short-term hospitals appeared more liberal than long-term, who range from 1 hour on Sunday only to unlimited visiting. In the short-term hospitals, the hours range from 1 hour daily to unlimited visiting. Of the 32 long-term hospitals, 13 have liberal visiting hours; 19 have restrictive hours. Of the 23 short-term hospitals, 21 have liberal visiting hours; 2 have restrictive hours.

14. RATING OF CHILD LIFE PROGRAMS BY OTHER HOSPITAL STAFFS

Various staffs in the hospitals contacted were asked to rate Child Life Programs according to four categories of understanding and acceptance: excellent; very good; good; and poor. Nursing service rated the highest number of programs —46; occupational therapy rated the lowest number—26. Of the staff 144 members—32 per cent—have excellent understanding and acceptance; 193—42 per cent—have very good; 100—22 per cent—have good; 18—4 per cent—have poor understanding.

	Excellent	Very good	Good	Poor	Total
		Understanding and acceptance			
Administration	15	22	5	0	42
Child psychiatry	16	12	5	0	33
Medicine					
Senior staff	12	16	7	3	38
House staff	11	13	9	2	35
Surgery					
Senior staff	7	8	13	1	29
House staff	9	10	8	2	29
Orthopedics					
Senior staff	10	12	12	5	39
House staff	9	10	8	2	29
Nursing education	8	18	5	2	33
Nursing service	16	23	6	1	46
Occupational therapy	9	11	6	0	26
Physical therapy	7	23	9	0	39
Social service	15	15	7	0	37
	144	193	100	18	

SUMMARY

The most outstanding characteristic of the replies to the survey was the extreme variation among hospitals both in their Child Life Programs and in their recognition of the need for such programs.

Of the 91 questionnaires used in the survey, 52 were answered by the hospital administrators. There were 49 long-term hospitals and 42 short-term. Of these, 69 reported Child Life Programs; 22 reported none.

Of the 91 hospitals, 53 provided detailed information on their formal education programs. There is 1 teacher for 8 children in the long-term hospitals; 1 teacher for 11 children in the short-term hospitals. Children attend school an average of 5.1 hours per day. Children's libraries are found in 52 hospitals; 13 provide budgets for them. Librarians usually work only part-time.

Specific information regarding recreation programs was provided by 45 hospitals. There is 1 recreation staff member for 22 children in the long-term hospitals and 1 staff member for 49 children in the short-term hospitals. Salaries for full-time personnel conducting Child Life Programs ranges from $2,300 to

$10,500 annually. In 24 hospitals such personnel have bachelor's degrees or master's degrees. Salaries for recreation personnel average from $5,300 to $5,400 annually. Those conducting education programs are almost always paid by local departments of education.

Student nurses are involved in 31 of the Child Life Programs. Almost half the student nurse groups both observe and participate. They are usually supervised by nursing personnel.

There are paid directors of volunteers in 33 hospitals. Of the adult volunteers 93 per cent are women; 7 per cent are men. Of the junior volunteers, 87 per cent are girls; 13 per cent are boys. There are 60 different volunteer tasks mentioned.

A total of 138 areas were used for Child Life Programs. Of these, 112 are playrooms which are open an average of 6.3 hours daily. The majority of the areas reported are used only for Child Life Program activities and average 1,145 square feet.

Mothers may live in at 21 hospitals. No more than 12 mothers live in daily in any one hospital. Charges range from none to $5.00 per day; physicians usually determine when mothers may live in. Visiting hours are more liberal in the short-term hospitals than in the long-term hospitals.

Other hospital staffs rated Child Life Programs favorably. Of these 74 per cent have excellent or very good understanding and acceptance; 22 per cent have good understanding; 4 per cent have poor understanding.

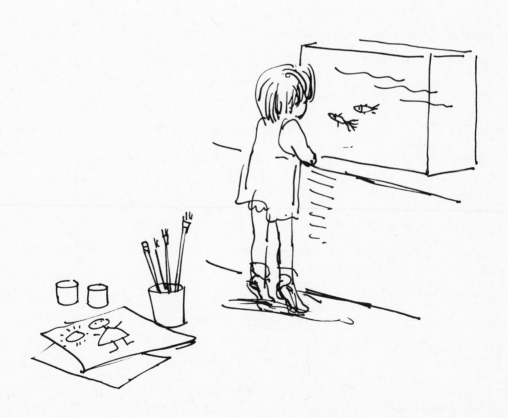

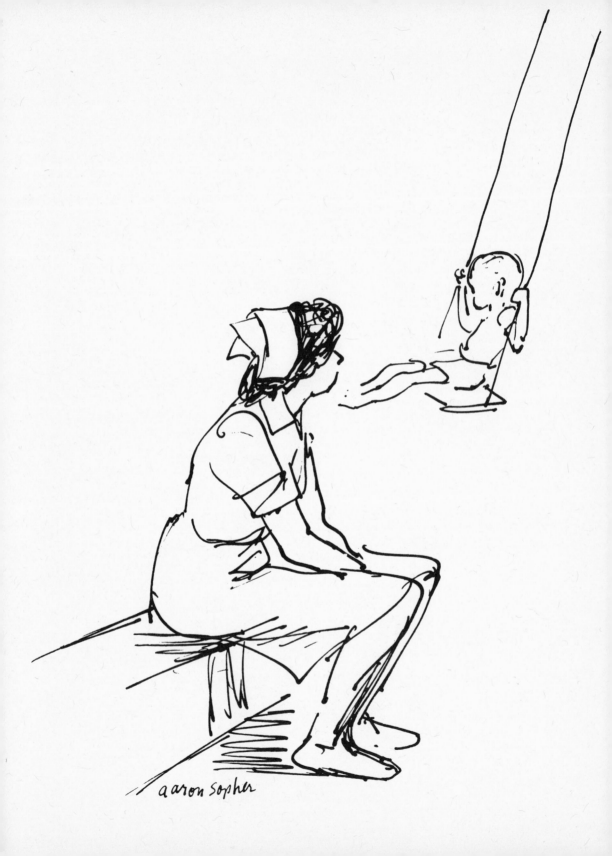

CHILD LIFE PROGRAMS IN NINETY-TWO PEDIATRIC DEPARTMENTS OF GENERAL HOSPITALS IN THE UNITED STATES AND CANADA

Robert H. Dombro, M.A.

INTRODUCTION

The 17-page questionnaire was also sent to pediatric departments of general hospitals with over 350 beds. Of 151 replying hospitals only 92—61 per cent—conduct Child Life Programs. Almost half of the 59 hospitals without programs do not feel the need for them; less than one-third desire to establish programs. There is a long list of program names and an equally varied administrative placement among the general hospital programs. The teacher-pupil ratio is comparable to that in children's facilities. There are 16 librarians in 35 libraries, with more than 14,000 books to be cared for. The least desirable child-staff member ratio is 1 recreation member for 70 to 80 children; salaries of staff are not significantly different from those found in the children's hospitals. Thirty Child Life Programs are used to train student nurses; volunteers are supervised by salaried directors in almost half the responding hospitals.

More than half the hospitals have specific areas for children's activities and provide programs 5 days a week; almost one-fourth of these areas are utilized for other purposes.

Twenty-one of the pediatric departments have facilities for mothers to live in, and the daily census is from 1 to 15, close to the number reported by the children's hospitals. Less than one-quarter of the general hospitals restrict visiting hours to less than 4 hours daily.

Thirty people (or 6 per cent) of the hospital staffs rate Child Life Programs "poor" on the understanding and acceptance scale; 18 of the 30 are from the surgical service. Some 606 people—94 per cent—of hospital staffs in pediatric departments who were asked to evaluate the effectiveness of Child Life Programs had "good," "very good," or "excellent" understanding and acceptance of them.

This report is concerned with a survey of Child Life Programs in pediatric departments of general hospitals in the United States and Canada. 151—36 per cent—replied. Of the 151 hospitals, 92 conducted Child Life Programs.[1]

The survey also attempted to gain information about 14 areas:

1. Number of Child Life Programs
2. Names of Child Life Programs
3. Placement of Child Life Programs in hospital structure
4. Children and staff in educational programs
5. Hours of school per day
6. Children's libraries
7. Children and staff in recreational programs
8. Salaries of staff
9. Student nurse involvement
10. Volunteer participation
11. Space allotted for Child Life Programs
12. Mothers' living-in programs
13. Visiting hours
14. Rating of Child Life Programs by other hospital staffs

The questionnaire was answered by them:

Answered by		Per cent
administrators	37	40
nursing directors	13	14
pediatricians-in-chief	12	13
directors of Child Life		
Programs	5	6
medical directors	3	3
social workers	2	2
no signatures	20	22

Hospitals were classified as long-term or short-term; 12 hospitals—13 per cent —gave no indication of length of stay. Long-term hospitals accommodate children

[1] A total of 7,089 children were in 90 of the 92 hospitals when the survey was taken; 2 hospitals did not report their census. Sixty hospitals reported 2,102 beds for prematures, infants, and toddlers; 32 hospitals did not report number of beds for these patients. This survey was taken in February, 1966, and completed in November, 1966.

two weeks or more; short-term hospitals, two weeks or less. Of the 92, 4—4 per cent—were long-term; 76—83 per cent—were short-term.

1. NUMBER OF CHILD LIFE PROGRAMS

Of the 151 hospitals that answered, 92—61 per cent—have Child Life Programs; 59—39 per cent—have no program. The latter group explained the absence of a program as follows:[2]

25 do not feel the need
19 do not have sufficient funds available.
17 do not have knowledge in the field.
6 do not know how to find staff.
9 give other reasons.
3 do not answer the question.

Asked if they desired to establish programs, they replied as follows:

17 desire to establish programs.
25 do not desire to establish programs.
8 desire to establish programs possibly.
5 do not desire to establish programs at this time.
4 do not answer the question.

2. NAMES OF CHILD LIFE PROGRAMS

The names used to describe Child Life Programs are numerous. Of the 92 hospitals 46 reporting programs have a name; 46 do not. The 46 programs are designated as follows:[3]

Educational-Recreational Program	7
Play Program	7
Recreation Program	6
Play Therapy	5
Children's Activity Program	4
Hospital Teaching Program	3
Child Life Program	2
Play Therapy-Teaching Program	2
Different names	10

[2] Some hospitals gave more than one reason.

[3] The different names included: Children's Ward Association, Educational-Recreational Therapy; Friends of the Hospital; Pediatric Education Program; Play Program–Day Care Center; Recreation Therapy; School–Occupational Therapy; Special Education Program; Volunteer Services; Ward School; Play Program.

3. PLACEMENT OF CHILD LIFE PROGRAMS
IN HOSPITAL STRUCTURE

Supervision of Child Life Programs varies. The majority is supervised by the department of pediatrics:[4]

Supervision	No. of programs
department of pediatrics	28
nursing service	16
occupational therapy	14
volunteers	11
administration	5
social service	5
nursing education	3
autonomous	2
child psychiatry	2
no answer	9
county, city, or state departments of education	22

4. CHILDREN AND STAFF IN EDUCATIONAL PROGRAMS

All the 4 long-term hospitals reported specific details about their education programs; 19 of the 76 short-term hospitals[5] reported details; 5 of the 12 hospitals not indicating length of stay reported details.

	No. of children	Education staff	No. of children per teacher (average)
Long-term hospitals 4	233	25	9
Short-term hospitals 19	243	27	9
No indication 5	69	7	10

[4] Several programs were supervised by more than one hospital department. Other programs reported that the teaching personnel was usually, though not always, responsible to the local department of education; consequently, some personnel had dual supervision.

[5] Three other short-term hospitals reported education programs conducted according to census; 18 hospitals reported tutors but not number of children taught.

In long-term hospitals number of staff members per child ranges from 1 member for 5 to 10 children to 1 member for 11 to 15 children.

No. of long-term hospitals	*No. of children per teacher*
3	5–10
1	11–15

In short-term hospitals number of staff members per child ranges from 1 member for 1 to 5 children to 1 member for 21 to 25 children.

No. of short-term hospitals	*No. of children per teacher*
5	1–5
6	6–10
5	11–15
1	16–20
2	21–25

In hospitals giving no indication of length of stay number of staff members per child ranges from 1 member for 1 to 5 children to 1 member for 6 to 10 children.

No indication	*No. of children per teacher*
1	1–5
4	6–10

5. HOURS OF SCHOOL PER DAY

Of the 92 hospitals 29 replied to this question. Of these, 20 have formal education programs; 9 have tutoring programs. The daily average is 5.6 hours. Tutoring ranged from one hour three times a week to one hour five times a week.

No. of hospitals	*Hours of school per day*	*Per cent*
4	3–4	20
3	4–5	15
5	5–6	25
7	6–7	35
1	7–8	5

6. CHILDREN'S LIBRARIES

There is a total of 35 children's libraries in 92 hospitals—all 4 long-term hospitals, 26 of the 76 short-term hospitals, and 5 of the 12 hospitals that gave no indication of length of stay had libraries. The number of volumes ranges from 50 to 3,000. The 4 long-term hospitals report 2,500 books, an average of 625. Of the 76 short-term hospitals 21 report 7,525 books, an average of 358. Of the 12 hospitals with no indication of length of stay, 3 report 4,250 books, an average of 1,417. Of the long-term hospitals 1 has a library budget and of the short-term hospitals 4 have one; 20 receive donations and gifts, and 2 did not answer the question. Of the 12 hospitals with no indication of the length of stay, 1 has a library budget, and 4 receive donations and gifts. Of the long-term hospitals 2 have librarians (1 part-time, 1 full-time), and 2 have none. Of the short-term hospitals 14 have librarians (all part-time), and 12 did not answer the question. None of the hospitals with no indication of the length of stay have either a part-time or full-time librarian.

	No. of libraries	No. of volumes
Long-term hospitals 4	4	2,500
Short-term hospitals 76	26	7,525
No indication 12	5	4,250

7. CHILDREN AND STAFF IN RECREATIONAL PROGRAMS

Of the 7,089 children reported in 90 hospitals, recreation programs are provided for 1,359. Of these hospitals, 39 reported as follows:[6]

	No. of children	No. of staff	No. of children per member
Long-term hospitals 4	154	4	39
Short-term hospitals 27	792	37	21
No indication 8	413	16	26

In long-term hospitals number of staff per child ranges from 1 recreation staff member for 10 to 20 children to 1 member for 41 to 50 children.

No. of long-term hospitals	No. of children per staff member
3	10–20
1	41–50

[6] Of the 76 short-term hospitals 15 have informal or unorganized recreation programs; in 4, volunteers conduct recreation programs.

In short-term hospitals the range is from 1 member for 1 to 10 children to 1 member for 51 to 60 children.

No. of short-term hospitals	*No. of children per staff member*
3	1–10
11	11–20
8	21–30
3	31–40
1	41–50
1	51–60

Of hospitals with no indication of length of stay the range is from 1 member for 1 to 10 children to 1 member for 71 to 80 children.

No. with no indication	*No. of children per staff member*
1	1–10
2	11–20
2	21–30
2	31–40
1	71–80

8. SALARIES OF STAFF

Salaries for full-time personnel conducting Child Life Programs range from $2,750 to $8,320 annually. Personnel range from recent high school graduates to those with master's degrees in social work and several years' experience. There are personnel with master's degrees in 2 hospitals and with bachelor's degrees in 14 hospitals. Those directing the recreation programs are almost always paid by the hospital; those conducting the education programs are always paid by the local departments of education, and their salaries are determined by the salary scale of the local departments.

The following salary information is for personnel involved in recreation programs who may also have responsibility co-ordinating the education program within the hospital. Of the 92 hospitals, 27 provided annual salary figures: 10 gave a scale and 17 gave only one figure.

Scale	One figure
$2,820–$6,468	$2,750
3,600– 6,000	3,000
3,900– 5,200	3,500
4,420– 5,980	3,600
4,680– 5,400	3,660
5,000– 5,600	3,780
5,486– 7,124	4,000
5,500– 7,500	4,350
6,060– 7,356	4,555
6,700– 8,000	4,940
	5,000
	5,100
	5,200
	6,500
	6,500
	6,600
	8,320

The average annual salary for the 10 hospitals is $5,644; the average for the 17 is $4,786.

9. STUDENT NURSE INVOLVEMENT

Of the 4 long-term hospitals 2 report that student nurses are involved in Child Life Programs; 22 of the 76 short-term hospitals report student nurses involved; 6 of the 12 hospitals with no indication of length of stay report student nurses in programs. The length of time spent in the programs varies from 5 hours to 1 week. Several hospitals having no formal Child Life Programs involve student nurses and the children assigned to them in educational and recreation activities as part of total patient care. Of the 30 hospitals reporting student nurse involvement, nurses observe the program in 1; observe and participate in 12; participate in 9; 8 hospitals did not answer the question. In 9 of the programs student nurses are supervised by nursing personnel; in 11 programs supervision is provided by educational and recreational personnel; 8 hospitals reported that student nurses are supervised by nursing and educational and recreational personnel; 2 hospitals did not answer the question.

Special classes for student nurses include the value of play and play materials, the value of mothers living in, social group work techniques, psychological needs of the hospitalized child, use of arts and crafts, and growth and development. Assignments include a diary of the playroom experience, an oral case presentation, and reading and summarizing pertinent articles and books.

10. VOLUNTEER PARTICIPATION

Of the 4 long-term hospitals 3 have paid directors of volunteers; of the 76 short-term hospitals 30 have paid directors; of the 12 hospitals giving no indication of length of stay, 9 reported paid directors. One short-term hospital reported a paid director of volunteers exclusively for its pediatric ward. These 42 hospitals reported 733 adult volunteers annually:[11] 720 women—98 per cent—and 13 men—2 per cent. A total of 753 junior volunteers (Candy Stripers)—736 girls, or 98 per cent, and 17 boys, or 2 per cent—work in 19 of the 42 hospitals. The majority of junior volunteers work only in the summer. In-service training programs vary from none to 15 hours, with several hospitals reporting continuous on-the-job training.

There were 46 volunteer tasks mentioned:

amusing	handiwork	reading
art materials	helping with school	rocking
assisting with admissions	helping with homework	running errands
assisting with discharges	helping in O.T.	showing movies
assisting study hour	holding	singing
bathing	holiday programs	supervising play
bedside visiting	infant care	supervising mealtime
bicycle riding	knitting	telling stories
birthday parties	listening	transporting
changing beds	mail delivery	trips
comforting	music appreciation	T.V. watching
crafts	nurse's aide	walking
dramatics	painting	ward clerk
entertaining	picnics	writing letters
extra T.L.C.	playing records	
feeding	portering	

11. SPACE ALLOTTED FOR CHILD LIFE PROGRAMS

A total of 53 hospitals reported 100 areas designated for programs: all 4 long-term hospitals and 40 of the 76 short-term hospitals; of the 12 hospitals not

[11] These volunteers work exclusively with pediatric patients.

indicating length of stay 9 have space available. Of these, 54 are playrooms. Other areas are schoolrooms, porches, solaria, basements, roof playgrounds, outdoor playgrounds, and day rooms. Of the 100 areas 74 are open 2 to 12 hours a day, an average of 6.2 hours per day; and 26 do not have a time listed; 3 hospitals reported a 6-day program, including Saturdays; and 2 a 7-day program.

Of the 74 areas listing a time for activities, 42 have programing 6 hours or more; 32 are available 6 hours or less. Areas are never used without supervision in 17 hospitals, and are used without supervision in 37; 20 hospitals did not reply to the question. Of the 100, 67 are not shared with other programs, and 27 are; for 6 areas there was no information regarding sharing. The square footage for 76 of the areas ranges from 96 square feet to 15,000 square feet (an outdoor area) per area and totals 54,279 square feet, an average of 714 square feet per area. Of the 76 areas 24 have more than 714 square feet; 52 have less.

12. MOTHERS' LIVING-IN PROGRAMS

There are facilities for mothers' living in with their hospitalized children in 21 hospitals; none in the 4 long-term hospitals and 18 in the 76 short-term hospitals; 6 of these indicated limited arrangements available. Of the 12 hospitals not indicating length of stay, 3 have facilities; 2 of these 3 hospitals offer a limited service. The number of mothers living in varies from 1 to 15 daily. Costs range from no charge to $22.00 per day. One hospital charges $5.00 a day for the first 10 days and $3.00 a day thereafter.

Of the 21 hospitals with living-in facilities, 10 provide them for mothers of any economic level and 6 only for mothers of private patients; 5 hospitals did not answer the question. Whether or not mothers live in is determined by physicians at 6 hospitals, by mothers in 6, by the physician and nurse in 2, by the physician and mother in 2, and by the nurse in 1; 4 hospitals did not answer the question.

13. VISITING HOURS

There were 53 replies to the question on visiting hours: 3 from long-term hospitals, 42 from short-term, and 8 from hospitals giving no indication of stay. Visiting hours range from liberal—4 or more visiting hours daily—to restrictive—

less than 4 hours daily; the majority of the hospitals are liberal. Visiting hours in the long-term hospitals range from 3 hours a week to 7 hours daily; in the short-term hospitals, from 1 hour daily to unlimited visiting. The hospitals with no length of stay indicated reported a range from 2 hours daily to unlimited. Of the 4 long-term hospitals, 3 answered the question: 2 have liberal visiting hours; 1 has restrictive hours. Of the 76 short-term hospitals, 42 answered the question: 32 have liberal visiting hours; 10 have restrictive hours. Of the 12 hospitals with no indication of length of stay, 8 reported 7 with liberal visiting hours and 1 with restrictive hours.

14. RATING OF CHILD LIFE PROGRAMS BY OTHER HOSPITAL STAFFS

Various staffs in the hospitals contacted were asked to rate Child Life Programs according to four categories of understanding and acceptance: excellent; very good; good; and poor. Nursing service rated the highest number of programs —51; child psychiatry rated the lowest number—35. Of the staff 228 members— 43 per cent—have excellent understanding and acceptance; 122—22 per cent— have very good; 156—29 per cent—have good; 30—6 per cent—have poor understanding.

	Understanding and acceptance				
	Excellent	*Very Good*	*Good*	*Poor*	*Total*
Administration	27	8	6	2	43
Child psychiatry	19	11	5	0	35
Medicine					
Senior staff	18	9	15	2	44
House staff	12	10	18	4	44
Surgery					
Senior staff	9	12	15	2	38
House staff	9	8	14	8	39
Orthopedics					
Senior staff	11	9	18	1	39
House staff	12	5	15	7	39
Nursing education	24	12	9	0	45
Nursing service	28	14	9	0	51
Occupational therapy	20	7	9	1	37
Physical therapy	18	5	15	2	40
Social service	21	12	8	1	42
	228	122	156	30	

SUMMARY

Again the most outstanding characteristic of the replies to the survey was the extreme variation shown among hospitals both in their actual Child Life Programs and in recognition of the need and support for such programs.

Of the 92 questionnaires used in this survey, 37 were answered by the administrators of the hospitals. There were 4 long-term hospitals and 76 short-term; 12 gave no information regarding length of stay. Of the 151 hospitals returning questionnaires, 92 reported Child Life Programs; 59 reported none. Names vary greatly.

Of the 151 hospitals, 28 provided detailed information regarding their formal education programs. There is 1 teacher for 9 children in the long-term hospitals, 1 teacher for 9 children in the short-term hospitals, and 1 teacher for 10 children in the hospitals that did not indicate length of stay. Children attend school an average of 5.6 hours per day. Children's libraries are found in 35 hospitals; 6 provide budgets for them. The 16 librarians conduct library programs; 1 is full-time; 15 are part-time.

There is 1 recreation staff member for 39 children in the long-term hospitals and 1 staff member for 21 children in the short-term hospitals. The hospitals with no indication of the length of stay have a staff member for 26 children. Salaries for full-time personnel conducting Child Life Programs range from $2,750 to $8,320 annually. In 16 hospitals such personnel have bachelor's degrees or master's degrees. Salaries for recreation personnel range from $4,786 to $5,644 annually. Those conducting education programs are always paid by local departments of education.

Student nurses are involved in 30 of the Child Life Programs. Almost half the student nurse groups both observe and participate. They are supervised mostly by educational and recreational personnel.

There are paid directors of volunteers in 42 hospitals. One hospital has a volunteer director assigned specifically to the pediatric ward. Of the adult volunteers 98 per cent are women; 2 per cent are men. Of the junior volunteers, 98 per cent are girls; 2 per cent are boys. There are 46 different volunteer tasks mentioned.

A total of 100 areas were used for Child Life Programs. Of these 54 are playrooms. Of these 74 are open an average of 6.2 hours per day. The majority of the areas reported are used only for Child Life Programs activities and average 714 square feet.

Mothers may live in at 21 hospitals. No more than fifteen mothers live in daily in any one hospital. The charge ranges from none to $22.00 per day; physicians and mothers usually determine when mothers may live in.

Visiting hours are liberal in 41 of the 53 responding hospitals. Four or more hours daily were scheduled.

Other hospital staffs rated Child Life Programs favorably. Of these, 65 per cent have excellent or very good understanding and acceptance; 29 per cent have good understanding; 6 per cent have poor understanding.

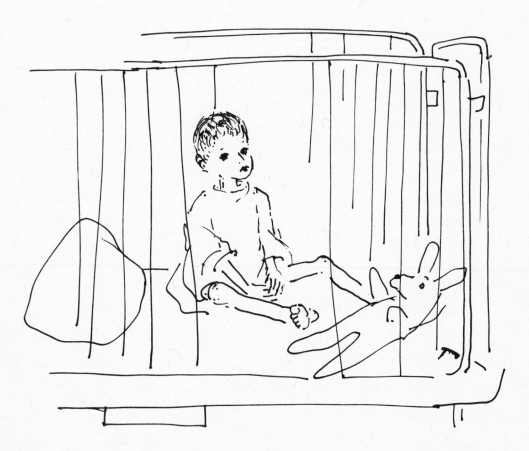

INDEX

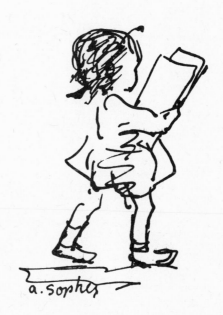

a. sophes

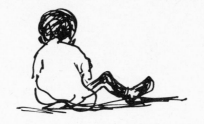

THE HOSPITALIZED CHILD AND HIS FAMILY

Editor: J. Alex Haller, Jr., M.D.
Associate Editors:
    James L. Talbert, M.D. , Robert H. Dombro, M.A.
Illustrated by Aaron Sopher

Designer:	Gerard A. Valerio
Typesetter:	Monotype Composition Co., Inc.
Typeface:	Fairfield
Printer:	Universal Lithographers Inc.
Paper:	60 lb. Offset
Binder:	Moore & Company
Cover material:	G.S.B. S/535 #95 natural

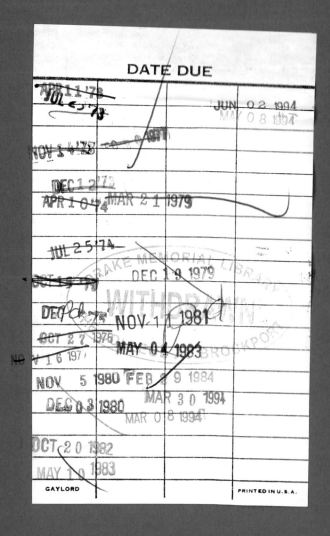

DATE DUE